Boatspeed

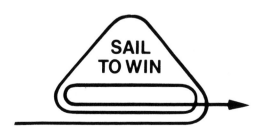

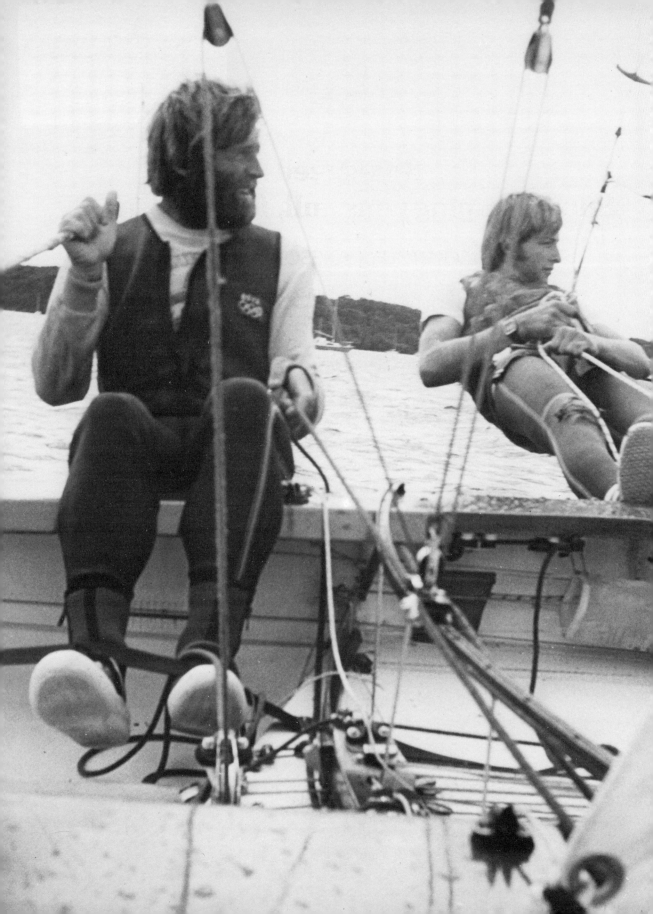

Boatspeed
Supercharging your hull, foils and gear

Rodney Pattisson MBE

with Tim Davison
photographs by Tim Hore

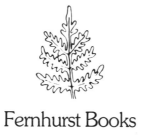

Fernhurst Books

First published 1986 by Fernhurst Books,
33 Grand Parade, Brighton, East Sussex
Printed and bound in Great Britain

ISBN 0 906754 25 9

Acknowledgements
The publishers would like to thank Tony Allen (of Holt Allen), the staff of Racing
Sailboats, Phil Milanes (of Milanes and White) and Lawrie Smith, for their assistance
with the manuscript.
   The cover photograph and the photographs on pages 6 and 19 are by Roger
Lean-Vercoe.

Composition by A & G Phototypesetters, Knaphill
Printed by Ebenezer Baylis & Son Ltd, Worcester

Contents

Introduction

This book is about putting together a boat that will win races.

It is perfectly possible to buy a second-hand boat and bring it up to scratch; indeed this may be all you can afford. In Chapter 1 I will show you how to assess an old boat, decide if it has what it takes, then supercharge it.

Alternatively, you may decide to buy new. In this case you need to be even more sure of what you want, so Chapter 2 covers each step of choosing and briefing a builder and checking each stage of construction.

A fast boat not only needs a good hull; each system must work properly. Nothing is more likely to kill speed than having to lean in and wrestle with a badly sited cleat, or trying to operate a control that has the wrong purchase. In Chapter 3 all the systems are studied in depth: the various methods of controlling rig tension, for example, are reviewed, giving the advantages and disadvantages of each. Where should you put the controls? How strong should the system be? What range of travel is needed? What about weight and windage? All these questions are considered, and conclusions drawn which will, I hope, help you choose and fit the best system for your boat.

Having put all this effort into getting the boat right, you will want to keep it in peak condition. Chapter 4 highlights a few ways to avoid deterioration, although major repairs are outside the scope of this book.

With a fast hull and rig and everything working properly you are ready to tune the boat and go racing – topics well covered in the other Sail to Win books (see last page for details).

So let's begin, as they say, at the beginning. Before you invest in a boat it is only sensible to do some spadework. Time spent analysing the class rules, talking to the experts and, indeed, sorting out your real objectives will pay handsomely later on.

Analysis of the class rules

Check first the materials that can be used in hull construction. Some classes can now use foam sandwich, which will revolutionise them. We will look later at the advantages of the various materials; obviously the right decision is vital.

Weight distribution is also a key factor. Check whether your class allows correctors, how heavy they can be and where they have to go. If you can put them in a useful place, a light hull with maximum correctors may be the best bet.

What tolerances are allowed on the hull? Originally, variations in measurements were allowed to help the builder: it was difficult to be a hundred per cent accurate, and without a bit of give and take no boat would have measured. But these days glassfibre boats are made in moulds and come out a very similar shape every time. This gives an opportunity to use the tolerances to develop a faster hull. Although we are only talking about a few millimetres, you'd be surprised what differences in speed can result. An FD, for example, should be built as wide as possible in

The author

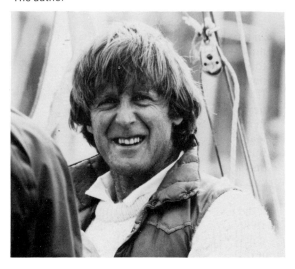

the forward section, then narrow at the next station, while giving a fair run throughout the boat. The straighter the waterline entry forward, the faster the boat goes.

The deck layout may or may not be limited; there are weight advantages in going for the minimum deck area. Similarly with the cockpit: see if you are allowed to have a double bottom or an open transom.

Having seen what the possibilities are, the next step is to find out what is currently winning.

Talk to the experts

The class measurer can be a fund of information. He is normally enthusiastic about the class and pleased to see a new owner. He will have seen a lot of boats and should have a good feel for what is fast: he may, for example, have measured the national champion's boat and know that it has maximum rocker – which may be the reason it goes so well.

Sometimes the class association can supply an analysis of what won where. Have a good look at this, bearing in mind that some crews are sponsored by manufacturers and have to use their products. Try to figure out why the winners chose a particular piece of equipment, and compare their crew weight and regatta venue with your own. If no analysis is available, make one up from race results and inspection of the fast boats.

You can also try talking to the experts; you have nothing to lose (they can only refuse), but be careful not to be misled. If you are told the opposite of the association's analysis, treat the information with suspicion.

Should you copy?

Many people try to use identical gear to the top boats. This is at least safe, but leaves them the task of outsailing the opposition on the water. If you are in doubt, or are new to a class – or intend to move class often – you have little choice but to copy the winners, allowing for differences in your own crew weight and the range of wind strength you normally encounter.

However, if everyone did this no class would develop, and no helmsman could expect to win. Imagine instead the confidence of going to a regatta with superior boatspeed. In the 1968 FD Olympic trials we decided to do something different and imported an Alspar mast from

Australia. The mast was thinner, stronger and had a better taper than the others in vogue at the time; but almost more important than making us faster, I believe it had great psychological effect on our opponents. I've no doubt that choosing a 'different' mast helped us win those trials and, eventually, the gold medal.

Objectives

Everyone needs an objective before he or she goes sailing. Yours may be to win the club series, an open meeting, or even a world title.

You also need a time-scale for your objective; your choice of boat will depend on how much of a hurry you are in. I was lucky in joining the Dutchman class early and being able to learn gradually. In fact my first boat cost only £220, and I worked really hard on it to save weight and develop the gear. Only when it became obvious that the boat was holding me up did I move on to the next one, and by that time I knew exactly what I wanted. The difference in performance was amazing.

Another advantage of starting with an old boat and time on your side is that you can change one thing at a time and see the effect of each purchase. This is an excellent way to learn – and you won't mind peppering an elderly hull with screw-holes.

New or second-hand?

Buy a second-hand boat if you are new to a class – for the following reasons.
- You may not be sure this is the class you want to sail. If you have to sell a new boat you will lose *at least* the cost of a new suit of sails.
- In a restricted class the probability of a newcomer picking the wrong design is just too high (but consider buying a new one-design).
- If you are a good sailor and have everything new you will expect to win, which is unlikely in a new fleet. It is better psychologically to learn in an old boat and improve gradually, buying better gear all the time.

Consider also the cost and time involved in working up a second-hand boat. If you have to redeck and realign the centreboard case, can you spare the time? Or can you afford to pay someone else to do it? In the end it might be cheaper to buy a new boat. Probably not – but do think about it.

1 Supercharging an old boat

Let's suppose you have decided to go for a second-hand boat. The first step is to find out the prices of a new hull and gear, otherwise you will be negotiating in the dark. You can do this either by asking a boat builder to quote for a complete boat, or by telephoning the manufacturer of each item. The expensive bits are, of course, the hull, mast and sails.

Finding a boat

Ideally, buy at the beginning of winter: prices are lower and you will have plenty of time to do up the hull.

Driving around to look at boats is an expensive hobby. Go to see the nearby ones to get a feel for the market; but use the telephone to check out the more distant boats before jumping in the car. Ask the owner the following questions.

- Who made the boat, and to what design?
- Which year was it built?
- Does it have correctors (i.e. can it be brought down to weight)?
- What condition are the sails in? Which loft did they come from?
- What state are the rudder and centreboard in?
- What type of mast does it have?
- Does the price include a cover, trolley and trailer?
- What is the boat's racing record?
- Is the price ONO, in other words is the owner prepared to negotiate?

If the answer to the last question is 'no', think twice about driving to see the boat because it is unlikely to be as good as described and you will almost certainly need to adjust the price. The description over the telephone is always better than the real thing!

If the boat does sound promising, telephone the builder to check on its history. "There are no correctors but I put a lot of timber round the case, which could be taken out" is a nice thing to know.

Now let's look at how to assess a boat and the amount of work needed to bring it up to to scratch.

The hull

The hull is something you are not going to replace, so take a long hard look at it. The paintwork and varnish will give a good indication of the amount of use it has had and the way it has been treated.

Look next for structural problems. Inspect:
- The mast heel area
- The shroud and forestay attachment points.
- The pintles.
- The centreboard case around the pivot bolt.
- Knees, frames and ribs.

Assuming the boat is sound, check its weight. (Reading the class rules will tell you if ropes and other gear should be included for weighing purposes.) You will need two bathroom scales; calibrate them with a known weight. Then put a polystyrene block on each, turn the boat upside down and support either end on the blocks. Adding the readings will give the weight of the boat to within a couple of pounds; however, ask when the boat was last sailed – a four-metre wooden boat may gain 4 to 5 kg by soaking up water, so the dry weight must be well below the minimum. Lifting the boat by its gunwales will give an indication of its centre of gravity – when you have done this to several hulls you will get a feel for where the boat should pivot.

Look for correctors (if in doubt, check the certificate – they must be recorded on it). You will be lucky to save more than 3 kg by drilling holes or removing paint, so correctors are a real plus.

The hull must be built true; to check this run a string from stem to stern and measure off the mast gate, shroud plates and so on.

You can assess the fairness of the hull as follows:
- Rub your hand over the bottom – you can detect minute imperfections down to 50 μm.

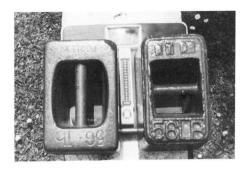

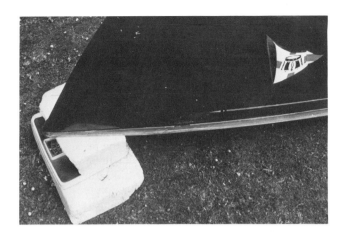

Calibrate your scales (above), then use them to weigh the hull (right).

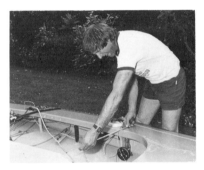

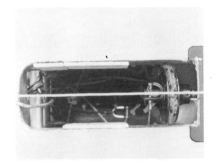

Run a string from the stem to the centre of the transom and ensure the boat is symmetrical about this line – in particular the shroud position (left) and the mast gate (right). Note the PTFE pads to hold the mast firmly while still allowing it to slide.

- Hose the boat down and look for bumps with the light across the hull. Note that imperfections on dark colours show up far better than on light colours.

Your hull needs to be as stiff as possible. Don't worry too much about the topsides, but press the pounding area (ahead of the mast foot) and the stamping area (floor of cockpit) to assess flexibility. Excessive flexibility can be cured by building extra ribs. If your class rules allow, these can be made of honeycomb sandwich (see page 16). You can stiffen the bottom in this way for virtually no weight at all.

Saving weight
If the boat is overweight you will need to do something about it. Here are ten options.
1 **Dry the hull**. Feel under the decks (the underside *should* be varnished). If they are bone dry, there is a good chance the hull is dry. If they feel wet, wash out the boat with fresh water (to remove salt) and leave to dry, preferably in a heated room. Then rub down and repaint, thus forming a seal to prevent the water being soaked up again. Note that two-part polyurethane is the only paint suitable for a wooden boat. If it is covered in conventional paint be very suspicious: you will have to remove the lot before painting with 'poly', otherwise the two types will react.

If there is a chip and the damp has got in you will have to go back to bare wood:
(a) Sandpaper back to the wood, tapering the edges.
(b) Apply undercoat mixed with thinner, so the paint gets into the veneers and grips.
(c) Paint on two normal coats of undercoat.

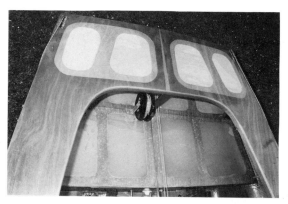

Mylar panels used to save weight in the deck and stern tank.

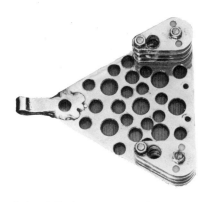

A bow fitting drilled out to save weight.

(d) After a few days, sand down.
(e) Build up with hard car-body filler.
(f) Apply undercoat.
(g) Rub down.
(h) Apply topcoat.
   Note there is no need to wait for one coat to dry before applying the next; in fact a second polyurethane coat seems to adhere better when the first one is still drying (but not tacky).
   There is normally no need to paint a wooden boat every year (you will only be adding weight).
2 **Remove screws** from glue-and-screw area, e.g. down the gunwales.
3 Provided you are not weakening the boat, **cut holes** in thwarts, knees and floorboards, and spokeshave deck beams. If the problem is acute and the class rules allow it, cut holes in the decks and use varnish to glue Mylar panels over the top.
4 **Change brass keelbands** for aluminium or nylon.
5 **Change stainless steel fittings** for aluminium, or even nylon (a stainless mainsheet track and centre jammer weigh a ton). Drill out metal where appropriate.
6 **Change to smaller diameter ropes** and use Kevlar or polypropylene instead of Terylene (they soak up less water). Taper sheets where possible: you can then substitute smaller blocks.
7 **Change mahogany to cedar** in non-structural areas.
8 **Replace rudder, tiller and pintles** with lighter alternatives.
9 **Replace bailers** with a lighter variety.
10 **Fit polypropylene toestraps**. These are light and don't absorb water.

Hull repairs

The style of repair depends on the material.

Repairs to glassfibre hulls
A hole is a specialist job.
   Hairline cracks in the gelcoat can be left. However, if the crack is structural it means there is movement at that point. It must be beefed up by adding glassfibre to the inside, or the hull may fail.
1 Fit a hatch (if necessary).
2 Dry the area and clean with acetone. Roughen with coarse sandpaper.
3 Mix resin and catalyst, and brush over the cracked area.
4 Place cloth onto the resin.
5 Dab more resin onto the cloth with the brush.

3 Using a knife, press in a mixture of microballoons and microfibres in a solution of epoxy and catalyst (don't use too much catalyst or the heat generated may cause a bump). When it is set, you will have a solid pad to bolt through.
and to keep out the air.
5 Dry for twenty minutes with a hair dryer, or leave it to set (one hour in the summer, one week in the winter).
6 Smooth off using wet and dry sandpaper.

Repairs to wooden hulls
A large repair (e.g. to a smashed gunwale) involves replacing wood: you will need to cut out the damaged piece and scarf in a new bit.
   Chips in the deck necessitate rubbing down to the wood, then applying several coats of thinned

varnish. Sadly, you will always see the repair.

A chipped hull can be repaired as described on page 63.

Repairs to composite hulls

Repairing honeycomb foam, carbon fibre and Kevlar is a specialist job, though for a small dent use filler as for wood. Remember that you can't sand Kevlar, so you will be left with an edge where it joins the filler unless you cut back the Kevlar with a surgical knife.

You can't screw into honeycomb. If you want to fix a new fitting to this material try to site it on a reinforced area. If this is not possible, reinforce the foam as follows:

1 Drill a hole where the fitting is to go.

2 Fit an Allen key to a drill and spin it between the glass surfaces to destroy the honeycomb in this area.

3 Using a knife, press in a mixture of microballoons and microfibres in a solution of epoxy and catalyst (don't use too much catalyst or the heat generated may cause a bump). When it is set, you will have a solid pad to bolt through.

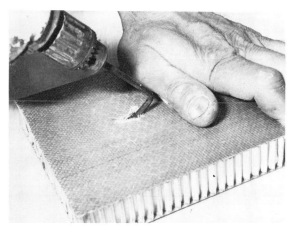

Above: drilling out honeycomb foam with an Allen key, prior to inserting microfibres.

Right: making a tapered sheet. (1) Use a thin and a thick rope. (2) Pull out the core of the thicker rope and cut off the last 15 cm. (3) Fuse the remainder of the core to the smaller rope. (4) Pull the cover down over the join. (5) Burn the frayed ends (6) Sew throughout the length of the overlap. (7) Sew around the join to ensure a smooth finish.

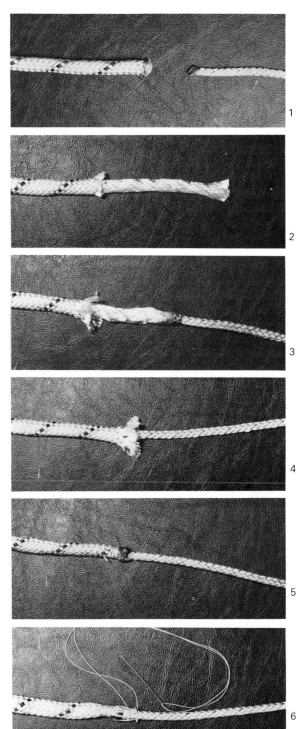

The centreboard

In this section I have relied heavily on the expertise of Phil Milanes (of Milanes and White, who make very fast boards and rudders), and thank him for all his help.

Check the board for straightness and absence of twist by sighting down each edge.

Roll the boat over, pivot the board down to the beating position and make sure it is a tight fit in the case by trying to move it about. You should feel no slackness (unless it is designed to angle when beating), but the board should still pivot. At the same time use the palm of your hand to check the board for fairness.

Stretch a string along the top and the bottom of the case to check that it is straight. Then jam a wooden rod vertically into the case and see if it aligns with the mast – if not, the case is leaning at an angle. The mast should have been previously aligned with the gunwales.

Construction

Wood (such as cedar, spruce or carefully selected mahogany) covered in glassfibre seems to give the lightest and strongest board. Carbon fibre can be used to great effect to stiffen it for virtually no increase in weight, (though it is expensive).

Section

A board is designed for efficiency on the beat and on a reach. In practice this is difficult to achieve, since the section presented to the water is quite different when the board is raised.

Let's look first at upwind performance. If the rules allow, the board should be shaped throughout, i.e. there will be no flat surfaces. For a boat that reaches off upwind and planes to windward, the maximum thickness should be 37 per cent of the way back from the leading edge. For a slower boat that points high, 30 to 33 per cent would be better. The figure for a gybing board is about 30 per cent. Note that this position of maximum thickness stays the same throughout the length of the board.

The leading edge must have a sensible radius – too sharp and it will stall after a tack, too blunt and it offers resistance at high speed. If the board is flat you will need a round leading edge to keep the water flowing onto the flat sections (otherwise laminar flow is lost).

The section should become very flat towards

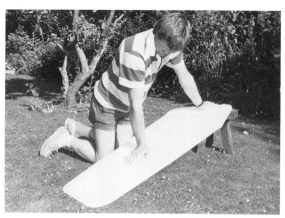

Checking a centreboard for stiffness.

the trailing edge (it would be no bad thing if it was concave here) and the edge itself must be razor sharp (any thickness, and the board will vibrate at speed). If you feel a sharp edge will get damaged, square it off so it is not more than 3 mm wide.

Note that if the section is wrong or the board is warped, nothing can be done with it and you will have to buy a replacement.

Shape

If the designer gave the boat too small a centreboard then go for maximum area; if it is too large, go for the minimum.

Everyone has his or her own theory about the fastest shape, but in general look for:
- Maximum depth, which is best aerodynamically.
- Maximum width at the top, to make this part stiff and to give power (which comes from area).
- Minimum width at the tip. The bottom 25 cm cavitate most of the time anyway, so you might as well reduce area (and drag) here.

Glider wings are often raked forwards and you, too, will get more lift to windward if the leading edge is raked forward slightly. It is possible that a board in this position takes up a positive twist under load, whereas a raked-back board twists the wrong way and forces you to leeward. At worst the leading edge should be vertical; raking it back is a last resort to keep the boat in balance in heavy weather. The angle of the trailing edge doesn't matter.

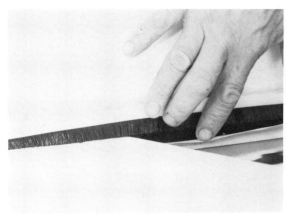

Slot rubbers made of draught excluder attached to an aluminium extrusion, with a Mylar sheet over the bristles to cut turbulence.

The profile near the bottom is important. A 'spitfire wing' shape has a lot going for it, since this gives an almost continuous leading edge. A board with a horizontal bottom edge would give too much resistance when raised for reaching, i.e. when the bottom becomes the trailing edge. For this reason the sections near the bottom must be flat and tapered.

Stiffness

A good centreboard needs some springiness. Just as a car without shock absorbers would be a disaster, something in a boat has to give as it smashes through the waves, or is hit by gusts. The best solution is a stiff hull and a board with a bit of give.

To compare the flexibility of boards simply bend them as shown in the photograph, or clamp them to a table and put a heavy weight near the tip. Ideally, the board should be very stiff around the case with the flexibility near the tip – in rather the same way that a mast is designed. A splice two-thirds of the way down, joining mahogany at the top to beech or balsa at the tip, will achieve this.

Twist in a board can be helpful if the leading edge moves up to windward (it then behaves like a gybing board). The configuration for this is shown in the diagram.

A new board will often work wonders for a boat's performance; it can give as big an improvement as a new suit of sails.

Slot rubbers

Slot rubbers are designed to stop turbulence (shown by water spurting from the back of the case). They *won't* stop water entering the case up to the waterline, but they will prevent a further build-up at speed.

I prefer to use Mylar rather than sailcloth. To fit the slot rubbers:
1 Cut two overlapping widths (6mm overlap)
2 Pull straight at both ends and punch holes for the keelband screws.
3 Make a Mylar cap for the front end; this should be slightly domed and designed so that the board butts firmly against it in the fully down position.
4 Screw on the keelbands to hold the slot rubbers in place.

On my boat I have a shaped piece of polystyrene foam which I push into the back of the case on a reach to exclude water and prevent turbulence. A piece of sponge is fixed permanently in the front of the case for similar reasons.

The rudder

The rudder should be as small as possible (to reduce drag) while still having enough area to let you steer in heavy conditions. There is much talk in books and articles about weather helm, but in my view you only need this to help you spot windshifts, and helm should be reduced to a minimum. Hydrodynamically, lift from the rudder is not important and is best left to the centreboard.

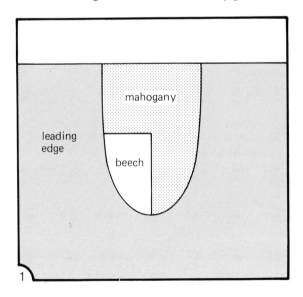

Lee helm, however, is disastrous, so don't overdo the tuning.

Section

Maximum thickness 33 per cent aft from the trailing edge is about right.

The leading edge should be round on boats like the Finn that are steered a lot, because the aim is to persuade the water to flow around the blade at enormous angles of attack. On a Dutchman the speed is higher so the entry can be sharper.

The trailing edge should be as sharp as possible.

Shape

The ideal shape for a rudder differs from a centreboard because the rudder is not raised offwind, therefore the bottom edge can be square.

A high aspect ratio is good; a deep blade gives more control on beamy boats where the rudder is lifted out of the water when the boat heels. If the boat is hard to steer consider a deeper or larger rudder if the rules allow it.

The width of the blade at the waterline is a matter for discussion. Some prefer a wide blade here to increase waterline length, even though turbulence is high due to wave generation. Personally I prefer the widest part of the rubber blade to be well under the surface.

Rake

Have a look at the rake of the rudder – ideally this can be varied, although it will usually be raked aft between 0 degrees and 5 degrees.

It is very difficult to steer accurately to windward if you have heavy weather helm. To counteract this the centreboard can be raised and/or the pivot bolt moved back. If this doesn't do the trick (or the rules limit the pivot position), rake the rudder further forward – though the leading edge should *not* go forward of vertical.

In light winds you may need to rake the rudder aft to gain more feel.

Repairing the foils

Any chipped edges must be repaired. For a small nick, proceed as follows:
1 Sand away the rough paint.
2 Paint with thinned polyurethane to seal the surface: filler will stick well to this.

3 Apply plastic padding, using the hardest type available.
4 Sand off using a block.
   For larger repairs:
1 Chamfer away both sides of the break.
2 Drill holes and push in long brass panel pins dipped in epoxy resin. This gives the filler something to grip.
3 Seal the area by painting it.
4 Tape cardboard over one side of the break and surrounding area.
5 Lay the foil flat and work plastic padding into the hole and under the cardboard.
6 Sand off using a block.
7 Paint.

The sails

Sails are a subject worth a book in their own right. Here I want to concentrate on deciding if the sails that come with the boat are clapped out or not.

Colour is the first indicator. Dirty sails have usually had a lot of use (unless the owner sails on a muddy lake). It is impossible to wear out a sail without the appearance deteriorating.

'Feel' can tell you a lot. Try to decide if the surface of the cloth has broken down; if it has, the material will no longer be stiff. Yarn-tempered cloth is easiest to assess; it is so stiff that each crease leaves a line and gives the game away.

Check particularly the inboard ends of the batten pockets, the cringles at the corners of the sail, the headboard and the stitching.

You should by now have a good idea of the condition of the sails (and will probably have frightened the owner stiff). There is little point in hoisting the sails to check on shape, because you can't tell if they are fast until you race. Bear in mind that you can always alter a sail if the cloth is OK.

The mast

Make sure the foot tenon is a tight fit in both the mast and the mast step. Check the spreader bracket carefully – it should be solid and have a reasonable bearing area, otherwise it may dent the mast.

Look for cracks in high-stress areas: at the heel fitting, vang attachment and shroud attachment.

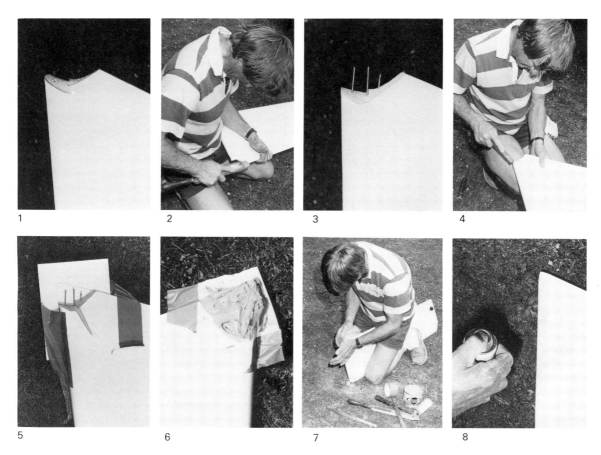

Repairing a damaged foil (1). (2) File the sides to a V. (3) Drill holes and insert panel pins and epoxy. (4) Roughen the surface. (5) Tape on a sheet of cardboard. (6) Apply plastic padding. (7) Remove the cardboard, then file and sand down (8) Spray on white polyurethane paint.

The sheaves for the jib and main halyards may be worn or broken, and the gooseneck bearing may be worn out.

Corrosion is a killer; look for it at boundaries between stainless fittings and the aluminium mast. Favourite points for attack are around the spreader brackets, the gooseneck fitting and the control line exits near the mast foot. To cure corrosion you will need to take the following steps.

1 Remove the fitting.
2 Clean off the corrosion with a wire brush.
3 Paint on zinc chromate to provide a barrier between the two metals (this chemical reacts with the aluminium to form a tough coating).

4 Replace the fitting.

If the mast is kinked you may be able to bend it straight, but be careful – you must work gently and try to reproduce (in the opposite direction) the force that bent it in the first place. It is unlikely, however, that your mast will regain the same characteristics, even if you do get it straight. In the Olympic trials one year we were limited to a single mast for the series. At the halfway stage our boat capsized, the mast hit the bottom and kinked. The committee refused to let us change it, but agreed to watch the next race. Our performance was dismal and very different on each tack; only then were we allowed to swap the mast.

2 Developing a new boat

Collecting a shiny new boat from the builder is one of the highlights of any sailor's life. Even better is discovering that your new boat is fast, and that most of the ideas you have poured into it really work. Genius, pure genius!

Unfortunately, as Thomas Edison noted, genius is one per cent inspiration and ninety-nine per cent perspiration. You will never get the boat you want unless you are sure about your objectives, communicate them to the builder, and follow up to make sure he is carrying out the plan properly.

This chapter is designed to help you formulate your objectives and translate them into a race-winning machine. If nothing else, once you have read it you should be able to persuade the builder you are not just another rich grockle, but know what you want and mean business. But please don't tell him you've got all this from me – some of my best friends are boat builders!

Wood, glassfibre or composite?
Your first decision is what your potential world-beater will be made of.

Composite means a combination of modern materials such as foam sandwich, carbon fibre, pre-preg and Kevlar. These are the best materials to build your boat from (if the rules allow), but are also the most expensive.

The advantage is that the strength/weight ratio is infinitely better than other materials, giving a lighter, stiffer hull (although collisions can result in more extensive damage).

The main disadvantage lies in the detailed planning required. With foam sandwich, once the outer skin is broken there is just paper inside! So the areas under fittings must be reinforced as the boat is built, joins between knees and skin must be beefed up, and so on. In short, the hull has to be engineered right, and built by someone who understands the materials. If that happens, the boat should be fast.

In case you are not familiar with exotic materials, here is a potted version of their qualities.

Kevlar is a super-polyamide (like an exotic form of nylon). Its molecules form elongated chains which can't be stretched. This gives high tensile strength (it can even stop bullets), but no give. When Kevlar breaks, it breaks.

Carbon fibre has an even lower elasticity but is more expensive.

Foam sandwich consists of two outer skins of glassfibre or Kevlar with foam inside. The foam is usually polyurethane, sometimes PVC. The further apart the skins are, the stiffer the material becomes.

Pre-preg consists of a reinforcing laminate pre-soaked with resin. This is laid down in a mould and the resin set either by heating or by addition of a chemical.

Microballoons come as a powder and are, in fact, tiny granules filled with air. They are mixed with epoxy resin, and trowelled onto an area to fill space without adding much weight. When set the material is soft and easily sanded, so microballoons are ideal for fairing the hull.

Microfibres are short strands of cotton. When mixed with epoxy and allowed to set a strong material is formed, which holds together well. This is ideal for repairing a hole, for example. But microfibres are not light; by mixing proportions of microballoons and microfibres together before adding epoxy a range of materials can be produced, from heavy and hard to light and weak.

Glassfibre on its own is heavier than wood and not as strong. You can't get stiffness from solid glassfibre; the only way is to add ribs.

The main advantage is that glassfibre is maintenance-free, and after misuse is easy to repair.

Glass/foam sandwich is probably *the* construction method of the future. Foams are becoming lighter, the strength being given by thickness rather than foam density.

Wood is stiff for its weight and easily repaired. No mould is needed, and it is cheaper than composites or glass/foam sandwich. However, there is always a shortage of skilled craftsmen who can build a wooden boat.

Choose your material as described in Chapter 1 – that is, by researching carefully what is allowed and what is winning.

How to choose a builder

Builders learn by their mistakes. So choose someone who has experience of working with the type of materials you have selected – you don't want to be the guinea pig. It is quite in order to ask for a list of his previous boats' successes.

If possible, choose someone nearby so you can supervise the building (or at least show an interest).

The first meeting with the builder

The best way to get to know the builder is to talk to him. At this stage he needs to know what you want, and it is helpful if you go armed with a diagram of the layout and where the main fittings such as the chute and shroud adjusters will go (systems are covered in Chapter 3).

On the other side of the coin, get him to tell you how he is going to build your boat. How will he stiffen the hull? How will he make sure the centreboard case is aligned properly and is warp-free? What about the inside of the case – can he cover it in Formica to prevent the varnish wearing through and the case swelling? What about shape: what have the previous boats from the mould been like, and how can this shape be varied for your boat?

Have a good look at examples of his work, particularly those using the materials you have chosen. In the case of composite, this is absolutely vital; indeed the boat may even need a designer. Ian Howlett, for example, played this role in the development of my latest FD. He specified different thicknesses of composite for various parts of the boat, and the builder produced a sample of each type. Ian checked these before building went ahead. That hull is *fast*.

The aim of all this is to confirm to yourself that you have chosen the right person for the job. Once you feel sure of this, sort out the price (you must have a written quote), the deposit and the delivery date.

So now your boat is under way. In the rest of this chapter I discuss the main objectives to bear in mind during construction.

Weight

Your builder should be able to tell you what weight the bare hull will be. Then you can make plans, bearing the following points in mind.

- Save as much weight in the ends as possible, because this reduces pitching in a seaway. Do *not*, however, sacrifice stiffness or weaken essential areas such as around the pintles and the stemhead fitting.
- Build the boat below weight. If the correctors are allowed to be in the right place, then have a light hull with maximum correctors. If not, then the correctors should be equivalent to the fluctuation in weight between the hull when dry and wet. (If the boat puts on 5 kg when wet, the correctors should be 5 kg.) Use surplus weight to beef up the centreboard case and the thwart since these are central. Heavy fittings can also be used in the centre of the boat.
- The best place for weight is around the pivot point. You can find this by watching boats in a seaway, or by videoing them in action. In an FD, for example, it is around the back end of the case.
- Similarly, weight is better located on the centreline than towards the sides of the boat.

How to save weight

1 Choose the lightest material to do each job. A wooden hull made from three veneers, for example, can be ground away to two veneers above the waterline at the bow and stern.
2 Use lightweight bulkheads, drilling holes where appropriate (and using plenty of varnish to seal the end grain).
3 Cut holes in decks if the rules allow.
4 Design structural parts with weight in mind. For example, T-shaped deck beams are lighter than triangular ones.

Stiffness

The objective is to make the hull as stiff as possible for a given weight, particularly:
- Ahead of the mast (the pounding area).
- Where you stand (the stamping area).

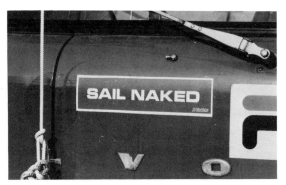

The final solution for weight-saving problems!

- Where the hull is flat (curved areas create their own stiffness).
  Stringers, ribs and foam sandwich can all be used to increase stiffness.

The centreboard case

The case is one of the most important areas in the boat.

- The overall objective is rigidity. The case must not move or twist, otherwise it will allow the board itself to move.
- Decide on the board thickness so the case can be built to hold it.
- If weight is critical certain parts can be light – the back end, for example, is only keeping out water.
- The points which support the board in the fully down position need reinforcing, particularly the pivot point and the area around the bearing surfaces at the back of the board. Beware of sandwich construction, which is not strong enough to support point loading.
- The case is well supported at the base by the hull, but the top edge needs capping with a wide strut to stop it twisting, and a beam (such as the thwart) to stop it moving bodily sideways.

However strongly things are built, they can still fail. One of my early boats had a solid mahogany case. After performing well for a long time it suddenly stopped pointing. I tried all the usual adjustments to spars and sails, but got nowhere. After a few more outings I noticed a small leak, which turned out to be a blessing in disguise as it

led me to discover a crack right through the case. A solid repair not only kept the boat afloat, but got it pointing again.

Beware of being carried away by your own zeal. One of my boyhood boats was a Firefly F27. To reduce its weight I spent hours substituting thin ply for parts of the mahogany case, and succeeded in removing a lot of timber. Only later did I realise the saving was more than offset by the extra weight of water the case now held, and the exercise was a complete waste of effort.

The deck

The construction of the deck can be treated separately from the hull.

- Construction must be of wood or composite. Solid glassfibre is too heavy, though glass sandwich is OK.
- Decks can be built very thin near the bow and stern, but need to be thicker where the crew sits.
- Decks must be varnished underneath (this is more important than varnish on top, as under-deck condensation is never dried by the sun).
- The tanks must be painted inside in epoxy.

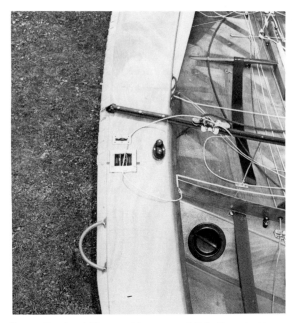

Gunwales should be as wide as possible in the crewing region. Note the footstrap to hold the crew aft on a trapeze reach.

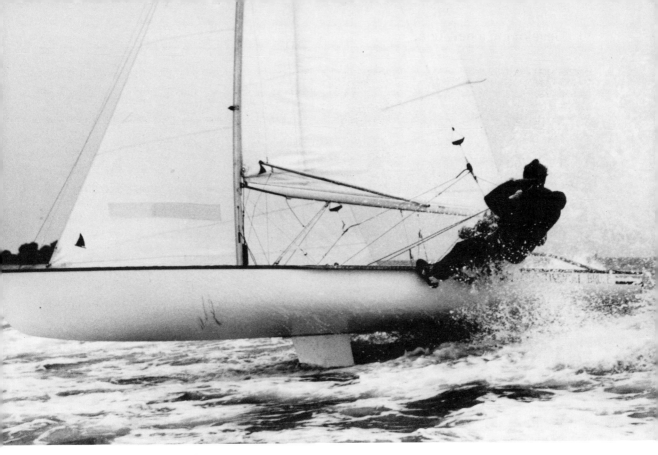

The correct centre of gravity is vital in a seaway.

- Hatches are essential for drying out the tanks, and should be sited so you can reach inaccessible points (your plan will have indicated where these are).

What to check before the deck goes on

1 Carry out a measurement check before the deck goes on. If anything needs putting right, now is the time to do it because the deck makes the boat rigid as well as inaccessible.

Use templates to make sure the boat is legal, and use a piece of string to see that it is symmetrical. Is the mast gate in the centre of the boat? Are the chainplates equidistant from it? Have a look at everything.

2 Make sure there are nylon tubes through the tanks to carry the control lines. If you have to lay these yourself, you can bend or straighten them by heating in boiling water. They should be sealed with a mixture of microfibres and epoxy resin where they go through the tanks.

Gunwales

In the crewing region:
- Gunwales should be as wide as possible for maximum leverage.
- They should be non-slip, particularly on a trapeze boat. You can either drill holes and thread a rope through or apply a mixture of epoxy resin and wood shavings.
- The outside 12mm should be of teak. This is comfortable and can take knocks without needing varnishing.

At the fore and aft ends use cedar wood or light mahogany (to save weight).

Intermediate measurement check

With the decks in place measure the boat again.

There is no point in working up a good hull finish only to wreck it with modifications.

Fairing the hull

The faster the boat, the more important it is for the hull to be fair. For a high-speed planing hull it is vital to have a really smooth finish. The method outlined here is ideal for a wood or glass boat.

1 Rub the palm of your hand over the hull to find small hollows, and ring them with a Magic Marker. Larger hollows can be found by laying a flexible 2-metre batten fore and aft along the hull and looking for gaps between them.

2 Rub down the hull with coarse wet-and-dry sandpaper (if you use it wet, you will have to let the boat dry before proceeding).

3 Fill major dips with soft car-body filler (e.g. Plastic Padding PP50).

4 Paint the hull with high-build paint.

5 Make a flat plywood board with a handle. Glue sandpaper to the bottom.

6 Sand fore-and-aft (and slightly sideways) because that is the way the water flows.

7 Check smoothness with your hand, or lay a ruler on the hull. Mark low areas.

8 Mix microballoons and epoxy resin and lay on with a spatula. When hard, use the sandpaper board again.

9 Put on two further coats of high-build paint, then sand smooth.

10 Paint on the final coats of two-part polyurethane.

11 Sand using wet-and-dry on a cork pad; only rub hard enough to get rid of brush marks. I usually leave the surface matt; but if you must have a shiny hull, buff up with polish.

Keelbands

Brass keelbands are easy to attach but are far too heavy for racing. Nylon strips are lighter, but can buckle in the heat. Wood is the lightest of all. If you are careful with the hull, wear-and-tear should not be a problem, but incorporate brass sections at load points, i.e. near the transom and where the keel rests on the forward chock of the trolley. To fit the keelband:

1 Drill holes in the keelband and push in panel pins.

2 Hammer the front pin into the hog.

3 Coat the underside of the keelband with polyurethane varnish (this doesn't dry too quickly).

4 Pull taut, and sight along the hull; then tap in the panel pins. In the centreboard region the keelband holds down the slot rubbers.

5 Fair off the ends of the keelband using soft car-body filler. Use the same filler to build a small dome on top of the slot rubber at the front end of the case. This gives a smooth flow over the centreboard.

3 Control systems

With the hull in good shape you are ready to start installing the various systems needed to control the gear. You will need to decide on a mast-rake system, for example, and then fit it to the best advantage.

In this section I look first at the various options for all the common systems, and then detail some general principles for attaching fittings to the boat.

The first five systems detailed below are used to adjust the rig, so it may be helpful to look briefly at why we need to alter mast rake, rig tension and mast bend while sailing. A fuller explanation is given in *Tuning Your Dinghy**.

Mast rake

Varying the mast rake can increase speed enormously, though no one is quite sure why. Rake doesn't help much on a light-air beat, but as the wind increases it pays to rake the mast back; on a 470 the tip may move through 30 cm. The jib halyard is normally used to do this: letting off the halyard increases rake. Ideally the slack is taken up in the shrouds at the same time. If you are not allowed to adjust shroud length, set them before the race, bearing in mind the first beat is the most

---
* Details of other books in the 'Sail to Win' series can be found on page 64.

important leg. Note that offwind you need to reduce rake as much as possible.

Having set the rig, the next thing to sort out is rig tension.

Rig tension

Rig tension controls the effectiveness of the spreader support and, to some extent, the jib luff tension – though in most boats this is best controlled by the mainsheet. In light winds let off the tension to let the jib sag. As the wind builds up, increase rig tension – the mast will bend anyway and you will need to take up the slack.

Offwind let off the tension, allowing the mast to straighten and the rig to develop power.

Mast bend

Mast bend fore-and-aft flattens the sail, and to some extent increases rake.

Sideways bend is generally slow, unless you have a large genoa; in which case allowing the middle of the mast to move slightly to weather can open the slot and depower the rig.

Fore-and-aft bend is controlled by chocks at deck level, by the vang and by the spreaders. Side bend is controlled by chocks at deck level, by spreader length and by lower shrouds (if allowed).

Now to the systems themselves.

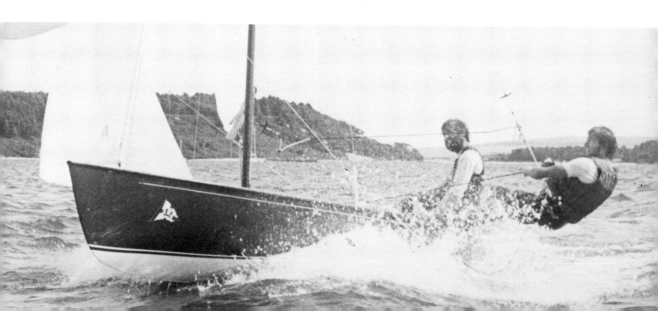

1 Mast

Go for the lightest, narrowest, stiffest section you can find. Unfortunately, these are conflicting requirements; you can't achieve stiffness without weight. And for a given weight, the larger the section the stiffer the mast. (In figure 2, A and B are of equal weight, but B is stiffer).

I believe windage is more important than weight in a dinghy because the boat is sailed upright. So go for a narrow section and accept the weight penalty to achieve stiffness.

Section

A poor section not only causes drag; it also ruins the airflow over the leeward side of the sail. Note that it is the thickness of the mast presented to the apparent wind when beating that counts (C in figure 3), and several ingenious designs have been devised to reduce this while keeping the mast stiff.

Taper

Turbulence behind the mast is a particular problem near the head of the main because there is no jib in this region to help the flow, and the sail is narrow so disturbance goes to half width or further. To minimise the turbulence, masts are tapered towards the top, which also saves weight where it does most damage.

Your spar maker should explain to you the method used to taper the mast, and you should be convinced this is satisfactory before buying. The section on construction that follows was supplied by Tony Allen (of Holt Allen), to whom I am most grateful.

Construction

Several methods can be used to manufacture aluminium alloy spars. Probably the first system, and one still used today, is adding a sail track to an extruded tube. The track may be an aluminium or even a plastic extrusion, attached by rivets, screws or glue.

The main tube can be tapered by cutting and welding: one or more long V-shaped pieces are cut out of the section which is folded until the edges are in contact, and the join is then welded along its length. Fore-and-aft bend can be increased by cutting V's from each side of the mast, while sideways bend is increased by cutting a V from the front.

Hammer swaging is another method of tapering, where the tube is crushed to a smaller diameter. A drawn taper mast, on the other hand, is manufactured by drawing the tube over a mandrel through an expanding die.

Any part of the mast can have its wall thickness (and therefore its stiffness) reduced by chemical etching or by grinding, and conversely parts that need strengthening can be sleeved or reinforced.

There is one other major manufacturing system,

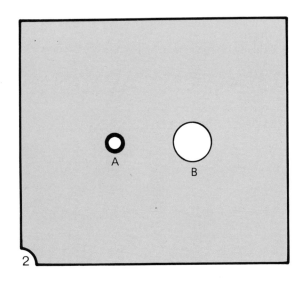

2

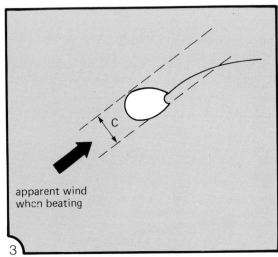

apparent wind
when beating

3

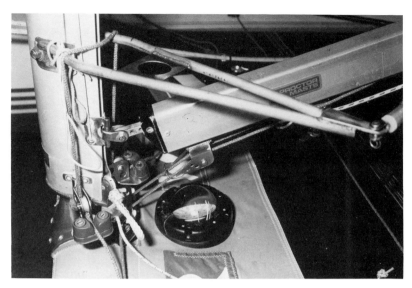

The rotating mast arrangement on a Tornado.

where the mast is made in two parts. The luff section and the front section are made separately with the fittings already riveted through, and any reinforcement or tapering is carried out before the two halves are glued or riveted together.

Springiness

Although the mast needs to bend, it must flip back quickly to its original position when the load is removed. I call this property 'springiness', and it relies on both the quality of alloy used and the heat treatment it has been given. Also a light mast with a large diameter will spring back quicker than a heavy one with a small diameter. (You can check springiness as described below.)

Choosing a mast

Despite all this, it must be admitted that choosing a mast is pretty hit and miss. Firstly look at the record of spars in the class, bearing in mind that heavier crews need stiffer spars, and select your section. Then evaluate several (supposedly identical) spars before picking the best:

- Support each mast at the gooseneck and hounds and hang a weight on it to give 75 to 100 mm of bend. Check the athwartships deflection. Twist the mast through 180 degrees and check it is the same in the opposite direction.
- Check the topmasts for deflection by supporting the masts in the same way but hanging the weight at the tip.
- Push down on each topmast to gauge how springy the mast is.
- Weigh each mast. If you are a bit heavy for the section go for the heaviest mast; if you are light, choose the lightest.
- Check that the masts are straight.

2 Mast rake

Mast rake is determined by the length of the jib halyard; the forestay is simply there for safety and is dispensed with in many classes. If you do have a forestay, fit a shockcord in parallel with it to keep the forestay taut and away from the jib roller.

Hooks

The simplest mast-rake system consists of a loop in the jib halyard which fits over one of a series of hooks. Unfortunately it is virtually impossible to alter·the setting while racing.

Muscle box

A muscle box on the mast takes up little room. There is, however, a lot of friction unless a ball-bearing system is used, and the range of movement is small.

Purchase system

A purchase system alongside the centreboard case works well provided ball-bearing microblocks are used. The problem is keeping the blocks clear of obstructions, so large holes must be cut in the knees. Alternatively, lead the system so the blocks run along the side tanks.

Winch

A winch is very efficient and very powerful. However, it needs to be supported by solid brackets and it is often difficult to find enough room for them at the foot of the mast. Use a shockcord to unwind the winch when the tension is released.

Calibration

Whichever system you choose, you must calibrate it. Put a mark on the control line (i.e. the line that leads from the blocks or winch to your hand) since this line has the largest movement. Fix a numbered track behind the mark.

Now we can alter rake we need a system to adjust the shrouds and thereby the rig tension (note that some classes prohibit shroud adjusters and the forestay is used for rig tension – though the rake is thereby altered too).

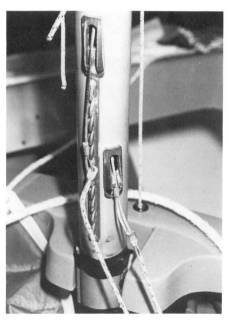

On a 420 you simply pull on the forestay and clip the jib halyard onto a rack.

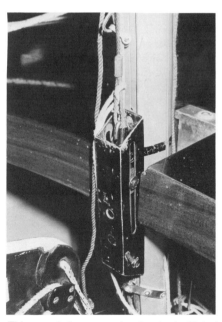

This muscle box controls rake via the jib halyard (FD).

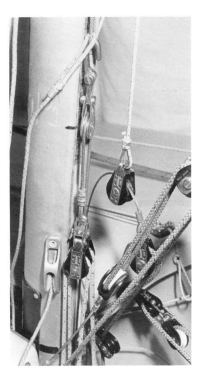

Here a simple block system hooks onto the jib halyard to control rake (FD).

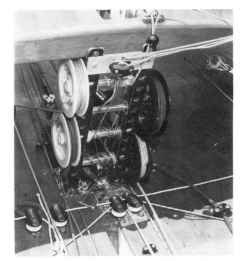

My FD has winches for many of the main controls.

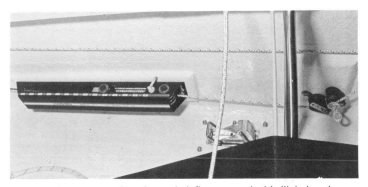

A muscle box mounted on the cockpit floor controls this jib halyard (505).

Forestay length is controlled by a hook on the jib halyard (left) connected to a block system (below). The shrouds are not adjustable when sailing (Fireball).

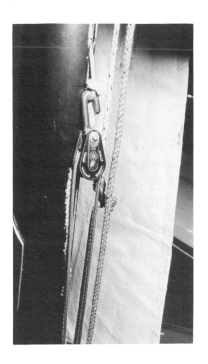

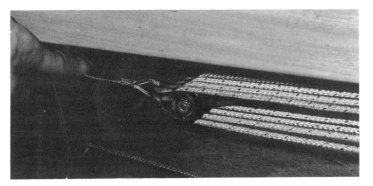

3 Rig tension

Rig tension is controlled via the shrouds. Note that if your class forbids shroud adjustment, you will need to use thick wire (1 x 19) or even rod rigging to prevent stretch.

Highfield lever
A Highfield lever is crude, and simply allows you to rake the mast forward on a run.

Purchase or lever
A purchase (as shown in the 505 photos) or a lever (International 14 photos) is more sophisticated.

Lever and tackle
A combined lever and tackle gives the best of both worlds. The tackle allows fine tension control (for speed on the beat), while the lever gives rapid rake alteration (when turning from a beat to a run).

Winch and lever
A combined winch and lever has the same effect.

Note that a rig tension system must be handed – i.e. both shrouds must be tensioned together, or the rig will lean over. In my early FD days I used to adjust the shrouds individually, but an excellent calibration system is needed to prevent a Tower of Pisa effect.

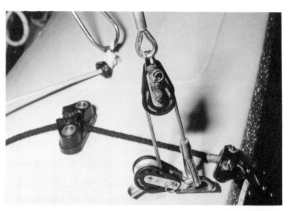

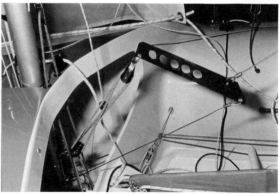

Right: rig tension controlled by wire and blocks; 2:1 at the shroud magnified by 8:1 near the cockpit floor, giving 16:1 overall (505).

Below: a simple shroud lever system (Intl 14).

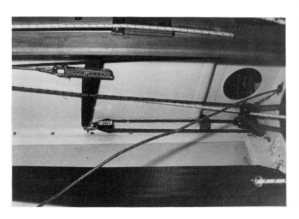

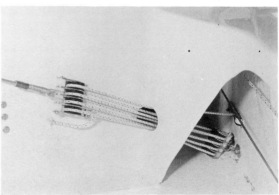

A more sophisticated set-up where a wire runs through the deck to the case and then to a lever, shown tensioned (left) and relaxed (right) (505).

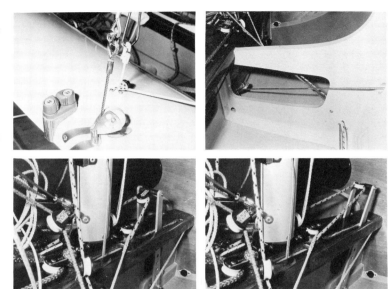

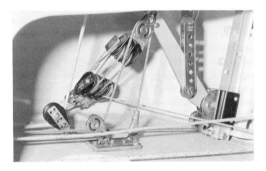

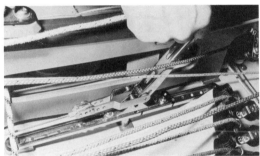

The lever/tackle system above is for fine-tuning the rig tension. There is also a coarse lever system which lets the rig forward quickly on the run (FD).

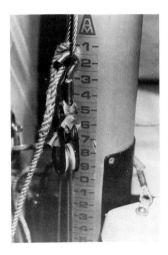

Right: a secondary system on my FD magnifies the shroud movement for calibration. It is repeated on the other shroud. Far right: rig tension via the jib halyard (470).

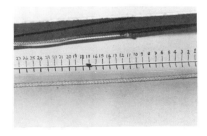

4 Spreader adjustment

It is now generally accepted that single spreaders in conjunction with gear to limit mast bend at deck level offer the best control for the least windage. Diamonds are not needed.

Bear in mind that spreader *length* (and shroud tension) control sideways bend. Length is not altered once you have got it right. In any case, angling the spreaders alters their effective length, so the system is self-compensating.

Spreader *angle* controls fore-and-aft bend. As the wind increases, more mainsheet tension is used, so the mast needs more support.

Holes

The simplest spreaders have one hole for the pivot bolt and you then drill another hole and feed a bolt through to limit swing. This is pretty hit-and-miss and weakens the spreader. It is also difficult to angle the two spreaders equally.

Screw adjusters

Screw adjusters are excellent, though they cannot be altered while racing. You can, however, adjust them between races by slackening rig tension and sending the crew up the mast.

Shroud tracks

Shroud tracks are fine provided the deck can be made strong enough and ball-bearing travellers are used. The system is not very 'clean' and is banned in some classes.

Spreader tip control

Here the shroud passes through a slit in the end of the spreader, and a wire strop pulls the shroud along the slit. The strop passes over sheaves to a muscle box or winch at the foot of the mast.

This system is becoming popular, though a lot of power is needed to overcome friction.

I think that the spreader tip system is very useful when you are using rake. If not, don't bother and use screw adjusters.

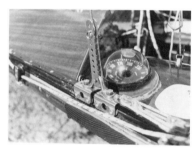

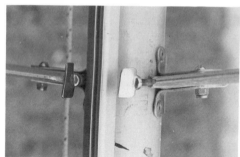

Top right: instead of adjusting the spreaders, the shrouds are moved on this 505. Right: screw spreader adjusters (470). Below: spreader tip control — wires run from the shroud to the front of the mast, then down to the cockpit (FD).

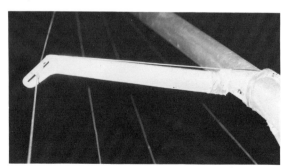

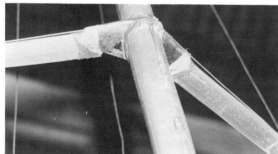

5 Mast bend control near deck level

If the gate is unrestricted (fore and aft) the mast will take up a smooth curve through the foot and hounds (which are fixed points). If you leave it like this:

- the mast may 'pant',
- the mast may bend too much;
- the mast may be bending in the wrong place for the cut of the main;
- there may not be enough bend for light airs. (In a zephyr, bend is best induced by the deck control rather than mainsheet or vang, which would also hook the leech of the main.)

The effectiveness of this control depends on the distance between the mast foot and the deck. If the distance is large, the control will be effective. If not, you may need to use a strut or even lower shrouds to maximise the height of the control.

Note that you may need to let off the tension downwind to straighten the mast. A run in heavy airs is not the time for the crew to be forward, so controls must be led aft.

Chocks

These are crude, but simple, cheap and light. They stop the mast bending but can't be used so easily to prebend it, and are not easy to vary during a race.

Wire and ferrule

A wire and ferrule system has similar advantages and drawbacks.

Screw

A screw at deck level is powerful, and can be operated from aft. However, it is slow to let off downwind, and hard to calibrate.

Right: chocks (Hornet).

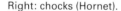
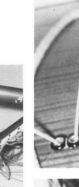

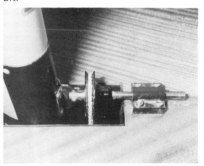

Below: screw (505). This is powerful, but unless the hole is elongated in the bracket the mast can't 'float' fore and aft.

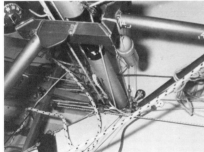

Above: this mast gate is supported by an aluminium frame (Intl 14). Right: wire and ferrule (470).

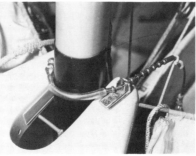

Strut

A strut gives control above deck level. The only way to organise this is with a track on the mast (a screw system, for example, is useless because the screw kinks, then jams solid). Although the strut causes windage and is expensive, it can be adjusted quickly and floats back immediately it is released.

Lower shrouds

Lower shrouds are very useful when the boom is high (to counteract boom thrust) or when the mast section is very whippy.

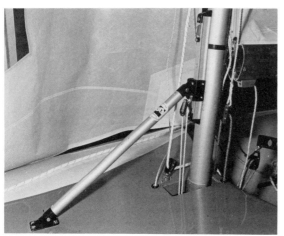

Strut (505)

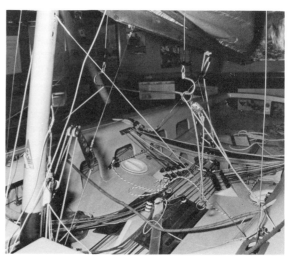

Lower shrouds led to a block system control mast bend low down (FD).

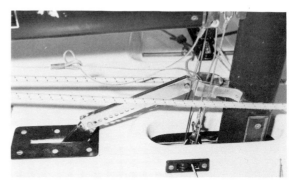

Lever (Star).

6 Mainsheet

It is best if the mainsheet is led from in front of the helmsman who can then tack facing forwards. In very small boats there may not be room, and the traveller will have to be on the transom.

Stern sheeting

This system is easy to install and gives room in the centre of the boat. But you can't jam the mainsheet, and it constantly pulls you inboard and aft. The weight of the traveller is right at the back, and it is hard to adjust. In particular, it is difficult to move the traveller block to windward in light airs to get the boom down the centreline and the leech open.

As the wind increases the traveller stops are gradually moved outboard. If you need to move the boom further outboard, vang tension must be used to prevent it skying. So the system is best for boats that are seldom overpowered.

Stern traveller with forward lead

A stern traveller with forward lead is similar, but allows you to tack facing forwards. A light boom can be used, because the mainsheet load is spread.

Hoop or strop

A hoop or strop means that the mainsheet only adjusts the athwartship angle of the boom. Movement up and down is left entirely to the vang, so a stiff boom is needed.

The system is simple, and gives a visual check on where the boom is in relation to the centreline (of course, the boom can't be moved to weather). When you tack there is no traveller to adjust, which makes one less job to do.

The main disadvantage of the hoop is that you lose the contribution of the mainsheet to preventing jib-luff sag. This is OK on a boat with a small jib (like a Fireball), where lots of shroud tension and pre-bend will do the job, but it won't work on a boat with a large jib or genoa such as the FD.

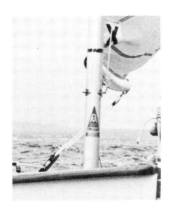
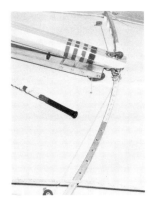
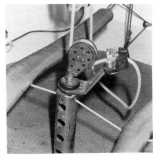
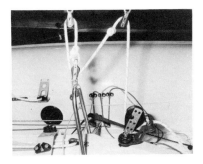

Above, left: classic stern sheeting (Enterprise). Above, centre & right: stern traveller with lead forward (Soling). Right: simple hoop (505).

Central traveller

A central traveller is my personal favourite. The track should be as long as possible for maximum movement, and set high to give more direct control athwartships – on my FD it is almost at deck level. Note that the mainsheet jammer needs to be as low as possible; with this combination the jobs of the mainsheet and traveller are kept separate – the traveller for boom angle, the mainsheet for leech tension. Personally I like to sail to windward with the mainsheet cleated, playing the traveller.

There is no need to curve the track, and a 2:1 purchase should be enough to let you adjust the traveller. Similarly, there should be just enough purchase on the mainsheet for convenience, but no more. So vary this according to conditions (e.g. 2:1 should be ample in light winds, while you may need 4:1 in a gale).

Mark the central position of the track. Otherwise, calibrating the traveller is not particularly helpful, because it is the balance between mainsheet tension and traveller position that you are after.

The main advantages of the system are positive control of the main's sheeting angle, and control of jib luff tension. The track also strengthens the boat, and keeps weight central.

The only real disadvantages are cost, obstruction of the boat, and difficulty in aligning the boom along the centreline.

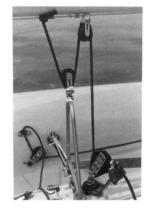
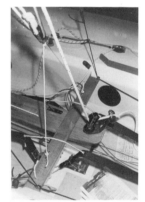

Near right: here the hoop is mounted on a traveller and the whole system can be moved sideways (470). Far right: simple strop (Intl 14).

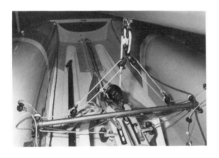
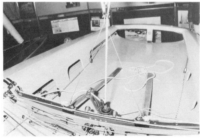

Far left: this adjustable strop allows the boom to be pulled to weather if need be. The strop needs to be shortened as the mast is raked back (470). Near left: here the ends of the strop can be moved (FD).

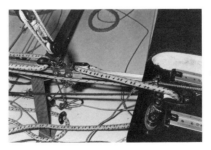
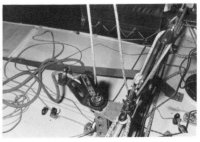

Right: classic traveller (FD).

7 Boom

Your boom should be light, stiff and deep. (Depth is important because it provides stiffness in the vertical plane, so that vang tension is transferred to the leech. Depth also increases sail area offwind.)

Initially it will pay to have an internal track so the take-off points can be varied. When you are sure of their position you can move on to a super-lightweight spar without tracks.

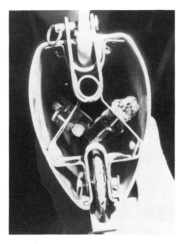

The inner workings of the boom (505).

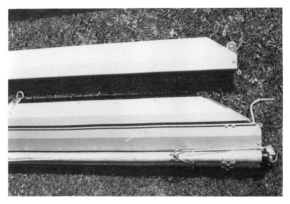

A normal boom section (top) compared with my deep boom, which gives extra area downwind.

8 Vang

The vang is one of the most important controls in the boat; it is essential to be able to alter it from either side. You will need at least 12:1 and possibly even 16:1 to be able to play the system properly.

Lever

The lever is a very clever, cheap and simple device. It can be attached straight to the mast (so organising the control lines is easy), and the power ratio is readily altered by changing the pivot point.

The main disadvantages are that the range of travel is limited, the purchase varies as the lever rotates, the system causes windage, and it may not count in the hull weight.

Although it is impossible to calibrate, you soon learn to judge the angle of the lever.

Winch

A winch is my personal favourite (see photograph). The system is very efficient, and the range of travel is unlimited since you can always put on or take off extra turns on the drum. The power is constant over the range.

The mechanical advantage is given by dividing the diameter of the drum by the diameter of the spindle. This can be lowered by sliding an aluminium tube over the spindle, or raised by incorporating blocks into the control line or the wire to the boom.

The winch is much better mounted on a stand rather than the mast, because the large forces involved will make the mast twist; even if the mast is held rigidly, wear will soon allow it to rotate. Also, when mounted on the hull the winch counts as hull weight.

The disadvantages of the winch are that the wire doesn't last forever (use flexible stainless wire); the system is difficult to organise (building the stand, and leading control lines to both sides); and the winch is bulky.

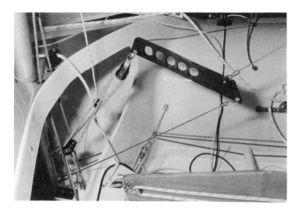

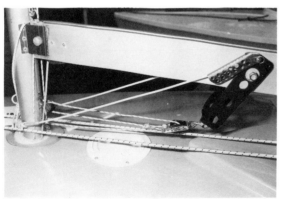

Levers (left 505, bottom left Finn, below FD).

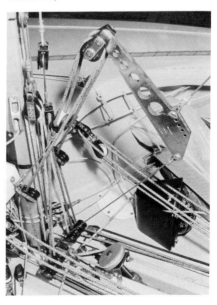

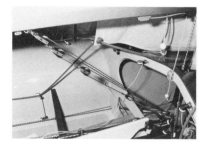

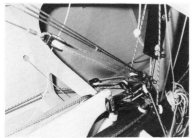

A 16:1 vang block system (505).

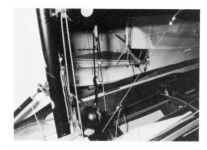

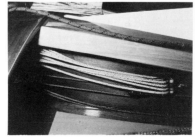

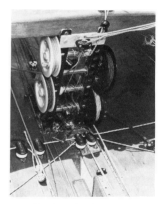

I prefer the winch
arrangement shown above.

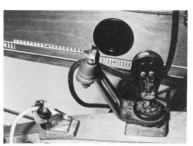

This vang is powered by a block system
and led to a mainsheet-type block so it
can be played on a spinnaker
reach (Fireball).

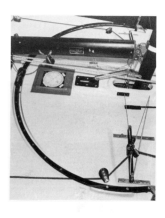

The vang track on a Star,
somewhat similar to a
mainsheet traveller.

Tackle

A tackle made up from ball-bearing blocks is
simple to fit, since all that's needed is a couple of
strong take-off points on the mast. It also has a
good range of travel.

Windage is a problem but can be reduced by
adding a strop so most of the system is below
deck level.

9 Cunningham

Not much power is needed on this control and 2:1 is usually enough; indeed the main problem is not pulling it on but letting it off.

To cut down friction the tack of the main can be cut away and a tape carrying a small block sewn to the sail. This is far better than simply passing the line through a cringle. The line itself can be very thin and a shockcord should be fitted to help the system relax.

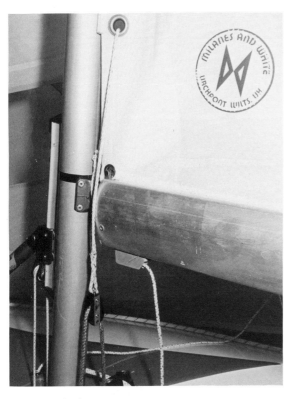

A 505 cunningham.

10 Outhaul

To counteract friction you need a lot of power to move the clew of the main (16:1 at least). Since you are short of space at the end of the boom, pass the outhaul rope through the cringle and then to a purchase system inside the boom or to a winch at the foot of the mast. A shockcord on the blocks or winch may help the system relax.

If the spinnaker sheet catches around the end of the boom, chaos ensues. To avoid this make sure the clew lies close to the end of the boom.

Also make up a nylon line incorporating a shockcord, with a hook on one end. Attach the line to the boom end and hook it to the leech of the sail.

In the Rome Olympics I was so worried about the spinnaker sheet getting caught that I fixed a glassfibre fishing rod to the underside of the boom, projecting well aft. The sheet caused no problems.

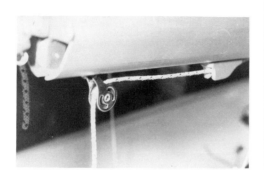 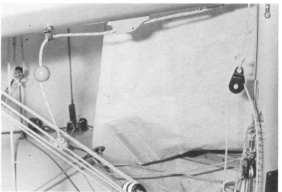

Left: an outhaul cleat near the mast, with the tail led through a block so it can be pulled by the crew in any position (470). The photograph on the right shows the same, but with the outhaul exiting the boom near the mast (470).

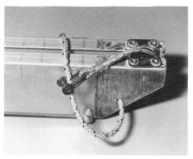 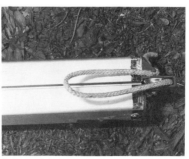

A 1:1 arrangement at the boom end (Finn) left, and right, a 2:1 arrangement (FD).

11 Jibsheet leads

Athwartships movement of the jib lead determines sheeting angle. Rather more important is fore-and-aft movement, which controls both the curvature in the foot and the leech tension: sliding the car forward puts more round in the foot and also tightens the leech, which is luckily just the combination you want.

Overall, as the car moves outboard it should also be moved aft, i.e. as the slot is opened the leech needs to be slackened.

Jibsheet tension also affects sheeting angle, foot curvature and leech tension. Ideally the lead should be as close to the clew as possible to counteract these effects: the idea is to make the sheet tension less critical so that the sail is set by determining the lead position, which can be done more accurately.

The range of travel fore and aft will need to be increased if you install a system for altering mast rake.

Positioning the lead

Positioning the lead can be very tricky because the deck or tank never seems to be in the right place. An FD and Star are fine, but a 470 has curved tanks just where the lead should go. The photographs show a couple of ways of getting round this, but the solution will always be a compromise.

If for structural reasons you really can't get the lead in the right place, you may need to use a barber-hauler. But this is a last resort, because the extra block increases friction when tacking.

In some classes, such as the 420, the lead position is fixed. If you want to alter the lead you will have to do it subtly – in the 420 pulling on the lazy sheet is the only way to close the slot.

The lead

For the lead itself use a ball-bearing sheave, not a fairlead, to cut friction when tacking. Note that a

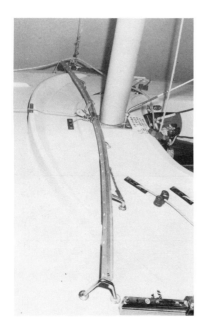

Self-tacking jib (Soling).

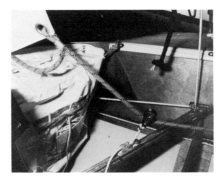

Left: vertical and athwartships control (Fireball). Below: this jib lead can be adjusted fore and aft and athwartships (Star).

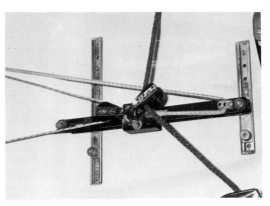

ratchet block on a jibsheet is a recipe for disaster, and many crews consider it unnecessary, even on an FD which has an 8 m² genoa.

The jibsheets should be marked so settings can be repeated on either tack: attach the sheets to the sail, stretch them equally and mark them together.

Athwartships track

An athwartship track gives excellent control of the sheeting angle, though this is not the most important adjustment. Fore-and-aft control is, obviously, limited; the only way to tighten the leech is by pulling the jibsheet harder, but this also tightens the foot, which is wrong.

A way round the problem is to tilt the track down at the inboard end (so when the slot is closed the leech also tightens) or to keep the track flat and angle it aft at the outboard end (which has the same effect).

Fore-and-aft track

A fore-and-aft track is better in that it can be used to alter the critical foot and leech tensions. It is a very positive arrangement.

The main problem is lack of athwartships control and you may need to add a barber-hauler for this.

Other arrangements

Other solutions to the problem abound. One of the neatest is the one Lawrie Smith uses on his 470. The lines and fixing points have been adjusted so that wherever the floating block is positioned it is self-compensating: the block moves outboard just the right amount when a gust hits.

The advantages are that operation is simple and as the leech is opened the foot is flattened. But siting is critical, calibration is difficult and the system is over-sensitive to jibsheet tension.

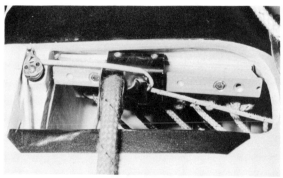

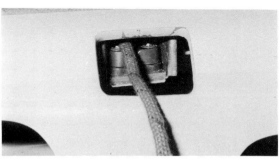

Above: sideways jibsheet adjustment (the gunwale is on the left). Fore-and-aft control by jibsheet tension (FD). The sheet then passes through the side deck to a cleat (lower picture).

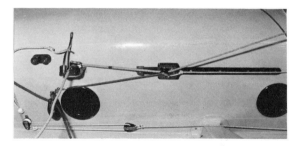

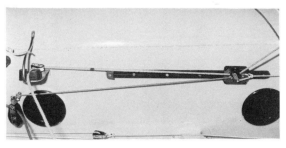

Above: fore-and-aft control on jibsheet lead. Note the tapered sheet and reference mark (470).

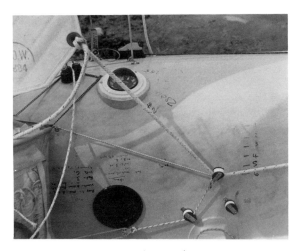

Lawrie Smith's 470 system (see text).

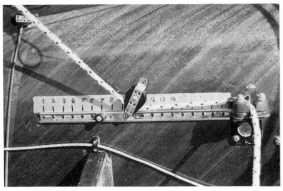

Fore-and-aft control on jibsheet lead. Note the calibration and carefully sited blocks (505).

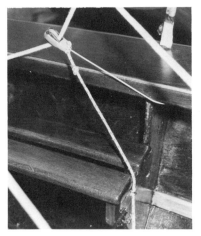

A very simple barber-hauler. Note the elastic to hold the block steady (Wayfarer).

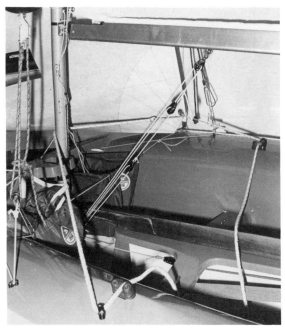

Using the lazy jibsheet to 'barber-haul' the clew to weather (420).

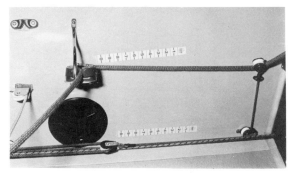

Jib leads with a barber-hauler led back to the helmsman (505).

12 Genoa roller

A genoa roller is very useful on the run to prevent the foresail interfering with the spinnaker. In light winds you may also need to roll up the genoa on a reach.

Ideally the roller should be below deck to reduce windage and the chance of fouling the kite. Also, the unwound genoa can fill the whole of the fore-triangle.

Although weight in the bows is critical, to work properly you will need a ball-bearing race at *both* ends of the jib. Tape up all the hooks so that it doesn't come undone when the genoa luff goes slack on the run.

A lot of string comes off the roller, and the line needs to be stowed properly – a drum at the back of the cockpit driven by elastic is ideal.

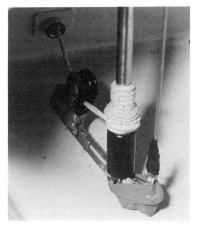

A genoa roller. Note the forestay attachment (FD).

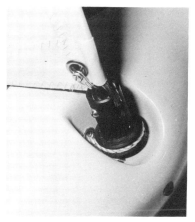

This genoa roller is faired into the chute (505).

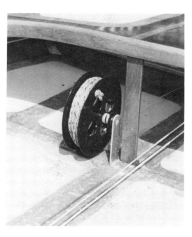

An elastic powered drum near the stern tidies the roller line (FD).

13 Centreboard hoist

When beating you can gain enormously by playing the board, raking it aft in gusts and forward in lulls. Not many people do this, however, because of the hassle of organising the system properly.

The problem is twofold. Firstly, friction on the board must be reduced. Wood-on-wood is hopeless – so either line the case or coat the board with Formica. PTFE on one surface and Formica on the other would be even better. Friction in the hoist is often a problem too; the lines must lead clear whether the board is up or down. Careful siting, ball-bearing blocks and Kevlar line all help here.

Secondly, the hoist almost needs two 'gears'. Enormous power is needed to move the centreboard a few centimetres when beating, but when you bear away onto a run only a small effort is required to retract it. The powerful purchase needed for the former means you have to pull huge amounts of line for the latter. A continuous system is clearly the answer.

Lastly, think carefully about the pivot bolt. Generally you don't need to adjust this while afloat unless you are playing about with the balance of the boat by altering rake. If you want the bolt to move you will have to plan this before the boat is built.

Standard 2:1 system
This is light and simple; but it rarely works well because of the lack of purchase. An improvement would be to have two tails to each line, one high-geared and one low.

The 4:1 system
The system shown here has the great advantage that you can lean in and pull sideways at points A and B (figure 4). 'Sweating' on the lines like this gives a huge purchase (perhaps 24:1). The system is continuous, too. With so many ropes running down the centreline it is essential to dye them so you know where to pull.

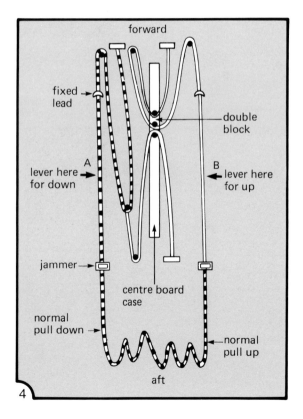

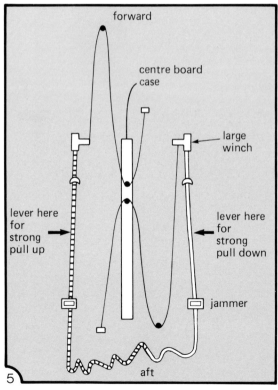

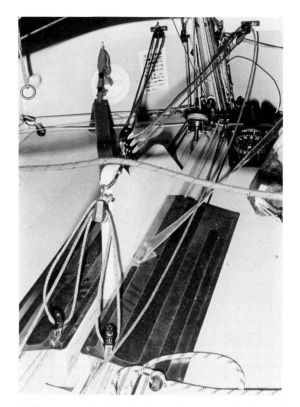

An FD system using blocks. Note the screw at the front of the case to alter the position of the pivot bolt; with it raised, the board area can be reduced in stronger winds.

Winch system

The winch system I use on my FD is possibly the best (figure 5). Wire is used virtually throughout so there is no stretch. The main worry is that the powerful winches may break their mountings, so they are fixed to special brackets. They also tend to be heavy.

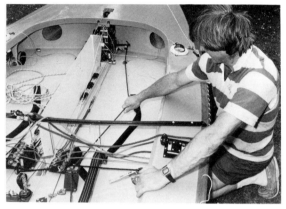

My centreboard system is identical to the one shown in figure 4. This action raises the plate.

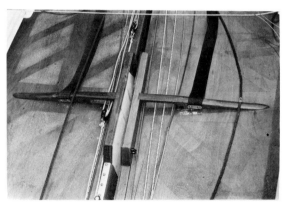

This case has Formica inside to reduce friction. Note the knee, which helps the case resist the loads imposed when the centreboard is right down.

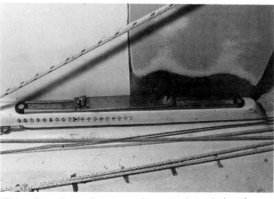

This stirrup is used to move the centreboard pivot fore and aft. Note the scale (FD).

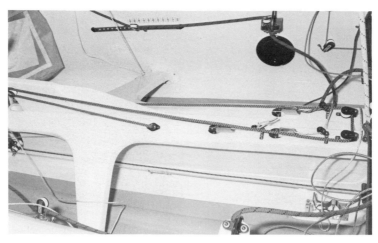

A simple uphaul/downhaul arrangement (470), and below on a 505.

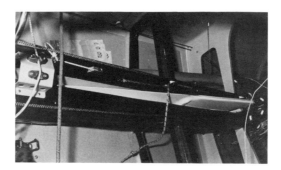

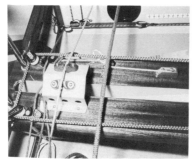
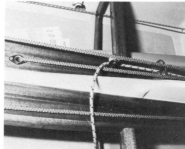
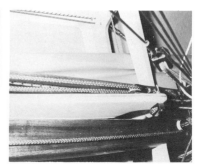

14 Trapeze

Your first decision is whether to go for a continuous or a separate system.

A continuous trapeze is quicker because the crew doesn't have to hook on or off. If you need two hands to handle a big genoa (as on the FD) this system is virtually essential. Problems will arise, though, if the boat is cramped: if the centreboard case or the vang restrict the crew's movements or the jibsheet leads are aft of the crew, the system won't work because it forces the crew to tack facing forwards.

The trapeze wires themselves can be thinner than the shrouds and are best fixed to the mast at the same point – this gives one less entry to the spar. But you may decide to attach the trapeze wires higher than the hounds to help support the topmast.

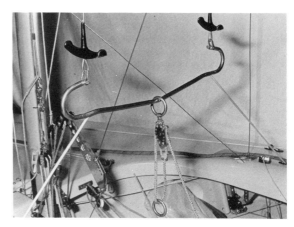

Continuous trapeze. With this set-up the system is inoperative if the shockcord breaks.

Continuous trapeze

The photograph shows how to organise the system. Note that the height of the hooks is critical (an alteration usually cures all ills). A handle is not needed, but a safety shockcord over the hook on the harness is essential to stop the crew coming off accidentally. The two sides are independent (i.e. the shockcord tails don't join up) so that if one breaks you can still sail on the other tack.

Separate systems

The ordinary trapeze system is now fairly standard but a few points are worth noting. I prefer a triangular handle to any other because it snags the jibsheet less. A two-position hook is good because it saves much adjustment between beat and reach (it also acts as a handle). A bowline at the end of the height-adjuster allows the crew to grip the tackle firmly for a good pull. Shockcord is always liable to break, so use Terylene line from the handle through the deck and shockcord as a tail thereafter.

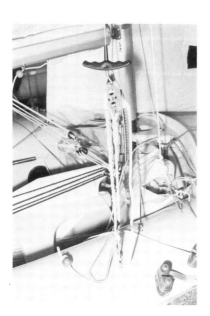

Left: a standard trapeze (470).

Below, left: a 3:1 trapeze control (Fireball); right, footrests for trapezing half-out (Hornet).

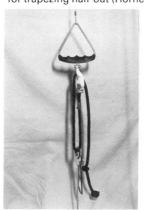

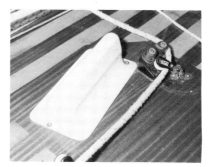

15 Spinnaker pole

Five systems are discussed below:
- Free pole.
- Double-ended pole stowed along the boom.
- Single-ended pole stowed along the boom.
- Self-launching pole.
- Double pole.

Your choice depends on three factors.

1 Your class rules.

2 The way you intend to gybe. The kite has a better chance of staying full if you don't end-for-end the pole, i.e. if you use a single-ended pole. Having both clews clipped on at the same time draws the leeches together and often results in a wrap.

3 The strength of your crew. A tall, strong crew can manage to push out the pole and clip it high onto the mast against the pull of the uphaul/downhaul. If your crew can't do this then a self-launcher will be better.

Free pole

In some classes (such as the 470) the pole fittings are limited to such an extent that the only system is a free pole stowed in the bottom of the boat.

The uphaul/downhaul has a hook which is attached to a loop on the middle of the pole, other fittings tending to detach during a gybe.

Double-ended pole stowed along the boom

Here the pole is pushed forward through a ring on the uphaul/downhaul. Provided you fit the right gate in the middle of the pole, you can end-for-end gybe.

Nothing is more distracting than the pole flopping around on the boom; arrange the uphaul block on the mast so that when the pole is set with its outboard end as high as possible, it can be released and swing back to lie properly along the top of the boom. Note that there is no elastic takeaway with this system.

Pole along boom with elastic takeaway

This is a very neat system, similar to the last one but requiring a single-ended pole. An elastic shockcord runs from the inboard end of the pole through a hole in the boom and then to a series of blocks. When the pole is unclipped it automatically takes up its position along the boom. When you gybe the pole has first to be stowed, then pushed out again from behind the main.

Self-launching system

This is similar to the previous system except that the pole is launched by a rope, attached at its inboard end and passing over a block on the mast. This means the crew need not struggle to clip the pole onto the mast fitting, but can stay on the wire while the pole goes out.

In my opinion it is better if the crew pulls the launching rope, otherwise there are times when he or she has nothing to do. Meanwhile the helmsman can be pulling the kite up or down.

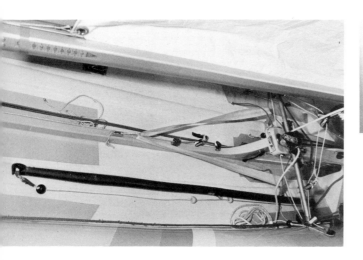

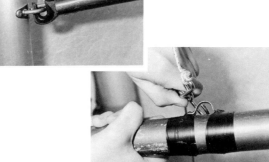

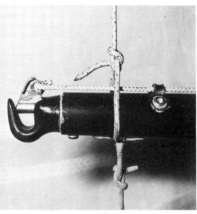
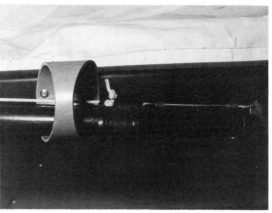
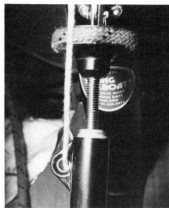

Single-ended pole stowed along boom. Note the downhaul passing through an eye in the strut.

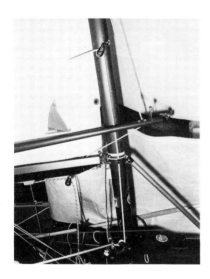
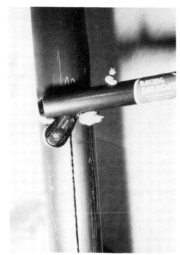
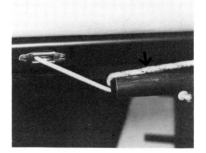

A self-launching pole system. Elastic holds the pole along the boom until the rope (arrowed) pulls it forward (Intl 14).

An elastic takeaway automatically stows the pole along the boom.

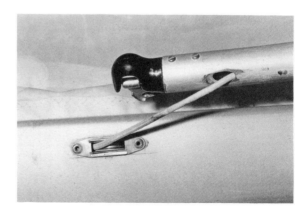

Opposite page: a free pole system. The uphaul/downhaul is clipped onto the middle (470).

Apart from weight and windage, there are no disadvantages provided the mast fitting is properly designed. If not, you will lose pole length.

Double pole

This system needs two poles, stowed along opposite sides of the boom. Each has its own uphaul/downhaul.

To gybe, simply stow the old pole, swing the main across and set up the new pole. The advantage of this method over the system with the pole along the boom is that the crew doesn't have to reach behind the main after the gybe to grab the pole.

The extra weight of two poles is minimal, and I strongly recommend this option.

Uphaul/downhaul

One of my earlier FDs had a double winch for winding the pole up and down, but really it was unnecessary. An elastic shockcord will do for the downhaul, because the guy pulls the pole down anyway, particularly when under the reaching

hook. But you do need an adjustable uphaul; this is usually operated by the helmsman and is led along the centreboard case to a cleat at the back. The helmsman can then lower the pole as the wind drops.

Should the uphaul/downhaul go to the middle or end of the pole? If you want to end-for-end when you gybe, clearly they should lead to the middle.

However, if the pole is long it is better to run the uphaul/downhaul to the end, because this bends the pole less. You may then be able to get away with a lighter pole section.

The pole

The pole itself must be light, stiff and strong. There is no need for a tapered section unless the pole is very long. Make sure the end fittings are compatible with the ring on the mast, which must stick out the maximum distance (this effectively lengthens the pole). The positioning of the ring is crucial: too high and the crew won't be able to clip on the pole and the bending moment will be large, too low and you lose effective length.

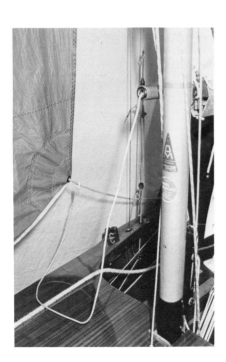

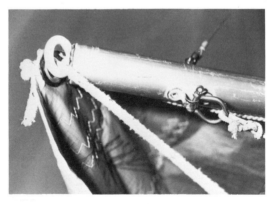

An alternative arrangement for a self-launching pole (Hornet).

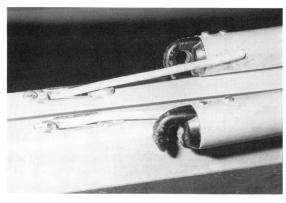

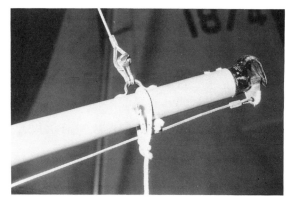

Double pole system. The inboard ends are pulled to the boom by elastic. The uphaul (wire) and downhaul (Kevlar) are attached short of the outboard end to make it easier to insert the guy in the hook (FD).

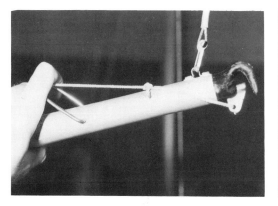

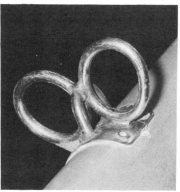

This handle allows for quick operation of the end fitting. It can also be operated by a line (FD).

These spinnaker pole rings are designed to maximise effective pole length (FD).

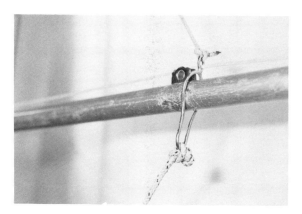

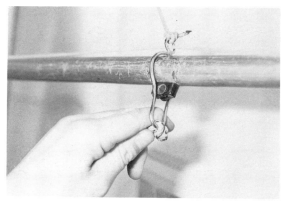

This uphaul/downhaul attachment allows the crew to gybe the pole end-for-end (Wayfarer).

16 Spinnaker sheet and guy

It is essential that the lines are tapered. This not only prevents the clew being weighed down in light airs, but also cuts down friction along the foredeck as the sail goes into the chute.

The lines must also be pre-stretched (Kevlar is best). Then when a gust strikes, the guy won't move and the pole stays steady. The last thing you want on a shy spinnaker reach is the pole to be blown onto the forestay.

The *lead blocks* should be positioned as far aft and as far outboard as possible to encourage the kite to lift. The only exception is when the boom is low and pushes down on the sheet; in this case you might as well have the lead further forward and lessen the friction of the sheet round the boom.

The *crew's lead blocks* should be placed so that the sheet comes straight across the boat to the crew's reaching position. Also the spinnaker and genoa sheets must not tangle, so it is best to keep the spinnaker lead aft of the genoa block.

Organising the system for reaching

The simple set-up described above is fine on a run, but extra gear is needed on a reach to keep the guy clear of the crew when trapezing.

The simplest method is to site a clam cleat on the deck just behind the shroud, with a hook in front. When the guy is under the hook it is automatically held in the cleat, which should be raised to help the guy in. A stopper on the rope enables it to be pre-set when hoisting or gybing.

A more sophisticated system uses a *twinning line* instead of the hook. This consists of a rope carrying a block through which the guy passes. When the rope is tensioned the guy is pulled down and into the jaws of the cleat as with the reaching hook (above).

The line must be pre-stretched (on my FD I use wire at the block end, with a rope tail); the whole point is to pull the block right down to the deck so the guy goes into the cleat.

The block must be as light as possible, otherwise when the twinning line is released on the run the clew will be weighed down. Once again tapered sheets help, because they need smaller blocks.

The position of the twinning line's cleat is not important; personally I prefer the crew to operate it, and avoid two ends by making the system continuous.

A stopper on each sheet makes gybing easier because the new guy can be pre-set. The only problem arises when lowering the kite – sometimes it goes into the chute unevenly and one stopper comes against its stop before the spinnaker is fully stowed. Indeed, the stopper may even prevent the kite being retracted far enough to keep it dry. These problems disappear if you use a detachable stopper that is clipped onto the new guy just before you gybe.

Below: simple twinning lines. Left, on a 470; centre and right, an FD.

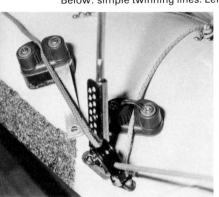
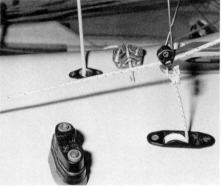
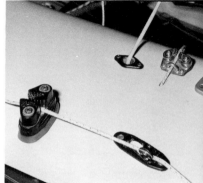

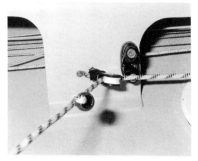 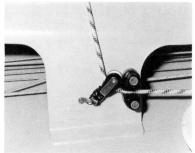

These cleats are so arranged that the jammer comes into play when the line is vertical (when it is the guy) but is not used when the line is horizontal (when it is the sheet). Note the stopper (left), set so the pole will be just off the forestay (FD). Below, a similar set-up on a Fireball (left) and a 505.

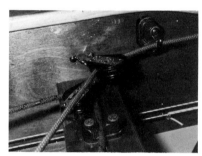 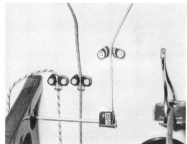

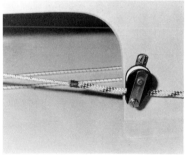

Tapered spinnaker sheet.

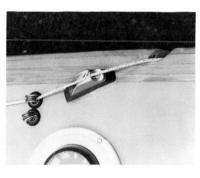

Left: I like the cleat close to the twinning line (FD).

Right: one method of organising the twinnning line control (505).

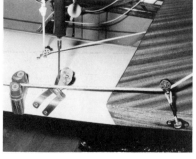 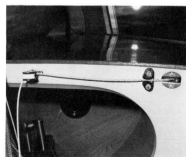

17 Spinnaker halyard, bags, retrieval line and chute

If the spinnaker is hoisted from bags the end of the halyard must be taken up on a drum or shockcord system. You can't risk coils of rope being loose in the bottom of the boat.

Use plaited rope for the halyard as this is less likely to kink, and make it of very, very thin line: this causes less friction through the mast, and less windage when the kite is down. Sadly, Kevlar is not suitable because it is not flexible enough round the blocks.

Fit ball-bearing blocks where the halyard enters and leaves the mast.

A fast-hoist system using a 1:2 or 1:3 purchase (i.e. you pull 1 and the halyard moves 2 or 3) gives a very quick hoist, though friction slows down the drop (shockcord can help here).

The bags should be made of netting (or at least have holes in the bottom) so water drains out; they should be as large as possible so the kite can be stuffed in quickly. Fit a waterproof cover over the top.

If the spinnaker is stowed in a chute, drainage is even more important to get rid of water before it gets to the kite. In most FDs the mouth of the chute runs through a bulkhead and there is a drain tube where they join. If you can't organise something like this, then a cover and drawline are needed.

Make the sock of netting or Mylar tube and have it longer than the kite so the sail will not be pulled into the cockpit, there to be trampled on or snagged.

The halyard and retrieval line are continuous. Find the correct length by tying the two ends together (with the kite removed) and trimming off excess rope. If you allow slightly too much rope you can then shorten the halyard when it wears around the sheaves. Remember to reverse the halyard well before it chafes through – this will double its life.

I prefer the halyard cleat to be out of the line of the halyard, so a positive action is needed to jam it. This prevents unwanted halts, and causes less friction when the spinnaker is lowered. Fit bull's-eyes every so often along the length of the cockpit to keep the flow going.

In fact my FD has two chutes so I can carry the normal-sized spinnaker and a storm or lightweight kite (depending on the expected wind strength). It is also a wonderful way of evaluating two kites, one after the other and before the conditions change. I use one hole in the foredeck and two netting socks, so the only real increase in weight is an extra set of sheets and their turning blocks. I reckon it is well worth it.

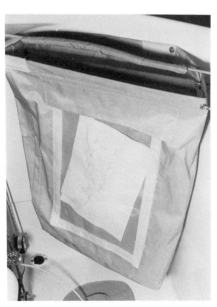

A spinnaker bag with a flap to keep the sail dry, and a pocket for race instructions (470).

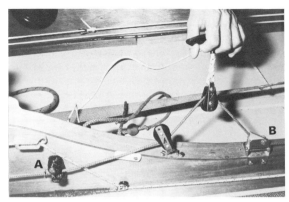

A pump handle on the spinnaker halyard. Note the cleat (A) and the swivel lead (B).

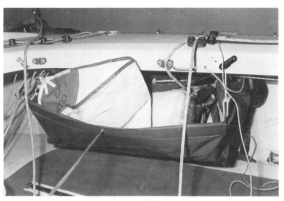

The spinnaker stowage on a Soling.

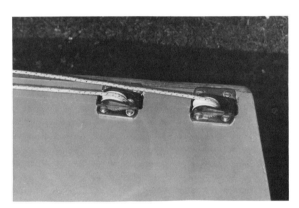

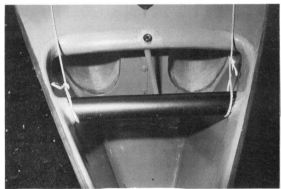

My FD has twin chutes, with two sheets and two guys. (These are prohibited for racing.)

18 Compass

A good compass should meet the following requirements:

- It should be large so that it is easy for the helm and crew to read. A dome gives good magnification.
- It must be well damped. Check this by turning it quickly.
- It is gymballed. Heel it to see if the card sticks.
- It has lubber lines such that both helm and crew can see them from their normal sailing positions.
- It has a temperature compensation device, or can be topped-up.

If your compasses are mounted on the side deck, tilt them outboard slightly so the crew can read them from the wire.

It is essential that both compasses read the same, or exercises such as taking wind bearings are meaningless. Align one compass fore-and-aft using a string down the centreline and measuring outboard with a ruler. Then go afloat (clear of any metal) with the second compass loosely in place, and swivel it until both read the same. Then screw it tight.

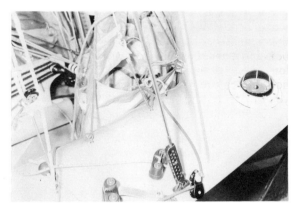

This compass is sited so the crew can read it (470).

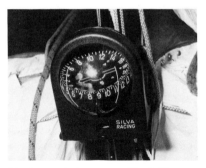

Mast-mounted compass (Fireball).

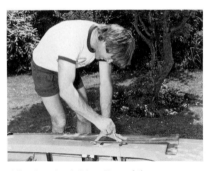

Aligning the lubber line of the compass.

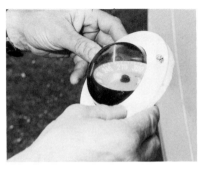

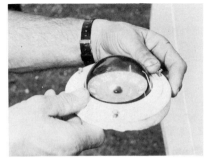

Checking the compass for heel (left) and spinning it to check damping (right).

19 Rudder and tiller

The *rudder* needs to be strong: there should be no play and no twist. Ideally, it should also be as light as is allowed, since it is at the end of the boat. A fixed rudder satisfies all these requirements, though you can't vary the angle of the blade, or raise it to clear weed.

The *tiller* is best made of aluminium. Although it may bend, it is unlikely to break like wood. The tiller should be short enough so you can squeeze between it and the mainsheet when tacking, but long enough to hold between your knees when hoisting the kite. If in doubt have it too long, as you can always shorten it.

It is difficult to get a tight fit between the tiller and stock, and a good solution is to have a Y-shaped end which fits around the top of the stock, and is then clamped on to it.

The *tiller extension's* length must be such that you can sit forward in light airs. You need a stop on the end. Criss-cross the rest with whipping twine and epoxy, for grip.

The *universal joint* is best made of rubber as there is then no angle at which it jams. However, the joint must stop the extension dropping below the deck (a good way to capsize, this).

The *rudder blade* has been discussed earlier. Paint it white (so that you can see weed – although in some areas the sea seems to be full of white plastic bags! Perhaps a black-and-white chequered blade is the answer). Arrange a stop to prevent the blade pivoting down too far, and rig a strong control line to pull it down. You will need at least a 3:1 purchase on this. Put marks on the line so you can see the rudder rake at a glance.

The *pintles and gudgeons* are best cast from aluminium – this is lighter and stronger than stainless, which can fatigue.

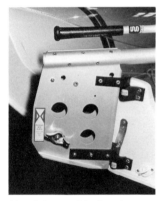

Aluminium rudder head (505), with tiller inserted.

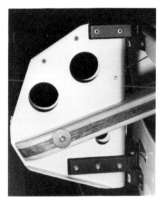

Tiller clamped outside an aluminium rudder head (470).

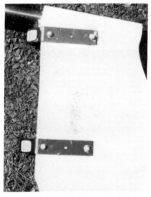

The fixed rudder on my FD. The gudgeons are of aluminium.

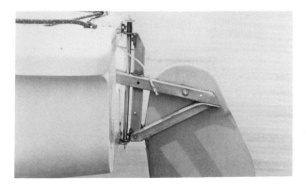

Left: an excellent lightweight rudder head incorporating the tiller (470).

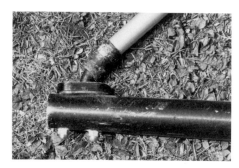

Rubber universal joint (FD).

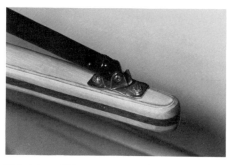

This joint will jam at some point.

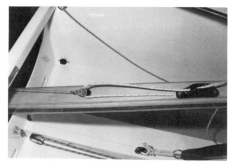

It is a good idea to have a purchase on the downhaul . . .

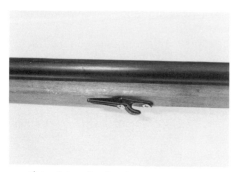

. . . though I prefer the cleat shown above.

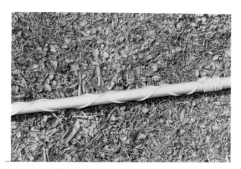

The tiller extension should be covered in glued-on whipping twine for grip along its whole length.

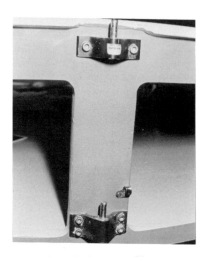

Aluminium pintles on an FD.

20 Bailers

One advantage of a double bottom is that you don't need bailers, the water simply going out through the case and transom.

All bailers cause drag, and you will go faster with them up. You may even need to restrict the swing so they don't protrude too far.

Fair in the bailer with plastic padding, not a rubbery filler which can't be sanded smooth.

I like to organise a system so I can raise and lower the leeward bailer with my feet, even when sitting on the weather deck.

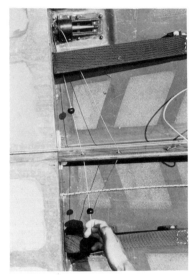

The bailers on my FD can both be raised or lowered from the windward deck by pulling the thin lines.

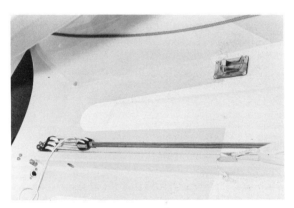

Bailer sited to remove water on the first reach (470).

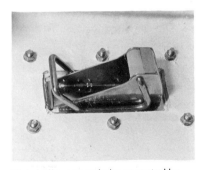

This bailer can only be operated by hand (505).

Attaching fittings to boats

Assuming you have made your choice for each of the twenty main systems discussed above, you now have to choose the right blocks, lines and cleats for each and bolt them firmly onto the boat in the right place. I hope the sections that follow will help you to do this.

Siting

The first question to ask yourself is: who is going to operate this control? In my opinion the crew should only have to adjust the jibsheet, spinnaker pole, spinnaker sheet and guy, and possible the twinning line (and these should all be calibrated so the helmsman can see where they are).

Everything else is best left to the helmsman: you are driving the boat and it is hopeless if you don't know the settings. Imagine going slowly, only to find the crew has altered something without your knowledge, or has tripped and accidentally moved a control line during a tack. Moral: lead the controls back to the helmsman.

Next, think about how often you are going to adjust each system. If it is constant use, and particularly upwind, you don't want to lean in every time; so the leads must come out to each side. Some things, however – like pulling up the kite – are best done in the middle of the boat. Occasionally it is impractical to lead certain control lines to the side: for instance, a centreboard hoist led in this way might mean your pulling 10 metres of rope to raise the board. In these cases run the control down the centreline.

Range of travel

A system has to cope with the complete wind spectrum; it is no good if you run out of travel when the wind blows up. Obviously the larger the purchase, the more the system has to move.

Strength

It is no good building everything too solidly: the systems should *just* do the job in the strongest winds you may encounter. Having small tolerances does mean, however, that you have to check the boat after every race.

Weight

All the fittings, bolts and screws taken together can easily weigh 12 kg, so you must choose them carefully. Weight normally equals strength, so choose fittings that are just strong enough for their job. On a dinghy aluminium will do unless the strains are enormous – such as on the spindle of a winch, which should be stainless. Remember that a drilled-out tube is nearly as strong as a solid one (provided the walls are not so thin they can be crushed), and the weight saving is enormous.

Correct lead

You should be able to get a near-perfect lead for each part of a system, particularly by using ball-bearing microblocks at each turn. If this is not possible, glue PTFE to any spot that rubs.

How well should it work?

Although a few systems (such as the cunningham) need not be super-efficient, most need enough purchase to work effectively when you pull them on. They should also run off when released; you can achieve this with shockcord, attached as near as possible to the moving part of the system.

Calibration

That great sailor Paul Elvström once said that nothing should be calibrated on a boat. While I agree that you can go badly wrong sailing by numbers, not many people have a perfect eye for sail trim: I certainly don't, and calibrate almost everything. After all, if you led at the windward mark you obviously went pretty fast; if conditions haven't changed you might as well begin the next beat with the same settings and *then* fiddle if need be.

Really it is a question of how you use the calibrations. Personally I note the settings in a book after a race. It is very interesting to study these during the season; maybe you won a race early in the year with one setting, and won again later on with a different set of numbers. Something must have changed; maybe the mainsail leech has stretched? Maybe the chainplates have moved (so the shroud tensions appear to have altered). In other words you can use the numbers diagnostically, in the same way that a motorist keeps note of fuel consumption.

If you are going to calibrate, site the numbers alongside the part that moves most (to give the greatest magnification). If this is not possible, for example on shroud adjustment, rig up an extra

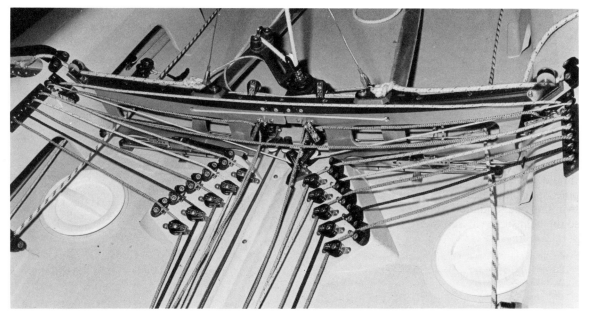

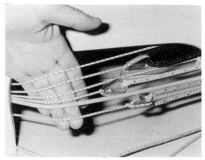
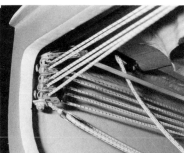

Tidying loose ends. On this beautifully fitted-out FD the cleats are near the centreline. The tails are taken through holes in the side deck to shockcords which run around the (open) transom to the tails under the opposite side deck.

purchase system so you *can* see what is going on.

Even if you don't mark everything, do calibrate the following:

- Main, jib and spinnaker sheets.
- Mast rake.
- Shroud length.
- Traveller.
- Spinnaker pole height.
- Centreboard up/downhaul.

Ropes and wires

If you have a long line that is stretching and causing problems, consider substituting wire. Wire stretches even less than Kevlar, although it

tends to kink and may jump off a block onto its axle. However, most non-winch lines on a dinghy tend to be rope.

Size of rope is determined by ease of handling, since the thinnest lines are so strong these days. Often you can taper them, making the working parts even thinner. On a 12:1 vang, for example, you can taper down to very thin rope indeed, since the line is only experiencing 1/12 the load.

Type of rope. Use pre-stretched plaited rope throughout. Three-strand is only suitable where you need to splice (for halyard tails, say) because it breaks down easier, knots, and is hard to handle. Kevlar is marvellous because it hardly stretches at all, but it doesn't like going round corners and this stiffness will cause friction. So for a pulley vang system it would be better to use pre-stretched.

If in doubt, you can pre-stretch your rope by tying it to something solid and pulling it behind the car.

Colour coding is essential: every rope of the same size should be a different colour. You will quickly learn to link a system with a colour, and grab it that much quicker. If you run out of colours, you can dye white rope as follows.

1 Put sufficient hot water to cover the rope in an old pressure cooker.
2 Add Dylon dye (use the whole container).
3 Add two teaspoonsful of salt.
4 Boil for half an hour.
5 Wash with cold water and hang up to dry.
6 The rope will have shrunk, so stretch it behind your car.

This is especially useful if you need different parts of a rope to be different colours, for example with a continuous centreboard control.

Tidying the end of every rope is vital. The method depends on the length of travel.

• For a one-metre tail, simply secure the end.
• For an intermediate length, use shockcord. If a simple length is insufficient build a shockcord purchase system. If the control is led out to each side deck, run one shockcord from the port tail, through blocks and back to the starboard tail.
• For a long tail such as the spinnaker halyard a roller is the best answer, though a shockcord system could be devised.

Simple tidying (Hornet).

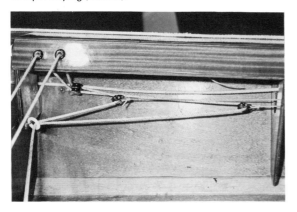

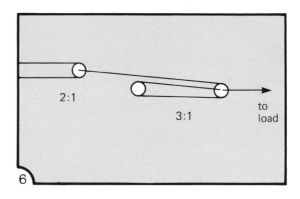

Mechanical advantage

You can work out the mechanical advantage (MA) of a block system by counting the number of ropes leaving the moving block. If there are three, for example, you have a 3:1 system.

If there is a further set of blocks on the tail, then multiply the two MAs to find the overall MA. For example, if the tail of your 3:1 system goes to a 2:1 block, the overall MA is 6 (2 x 3) (figure 6).

Cleats

There are three types of cleats:

• A clam cleat is like a tube with teeth. It takes up the minimum space, but the rope must be under constant tension or the tail can flick out of the cleat.
• A cam cleat has moving teeth. Set the springs so they just close the jaws (any more tension results in unnecessary work). As with the clam cleat, the load on the rope does the jamming.
• A 'standard' cleat needs the rope criss-crossed around it for security. Use this only when you need the rope to stay put with little tension (or when being jerked.) It has the advantage of allowing a rope under load to 'surge' around it and so is often used for mooring cleats.

The *bevel* on a cleat enables you to get the rope in with the minimum pull. The *teeth* must be sharp enough to hold the rope; to test, simply put in a piece of rope and pull! Plastic cleats always wear, and are best reinforced with stainless steel.

Choose a cleat as follows:

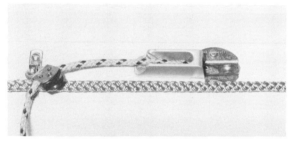

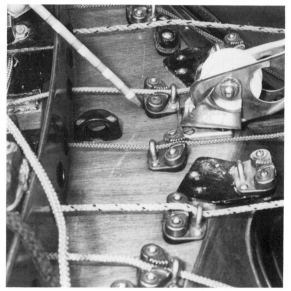

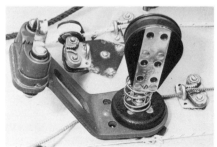

Top left: clam cleat. Right: cam cleats. Note the wedges, one of which is shown by the pencil. Left: the mainsheet ratchet block on my FD is held up by a spring.

1 The function determines the *type* of cleat (see above).

2 The load and amount of use determine the *quality*. For the cunningham you can use a cheap nylon job, but for the genoa sheet only the best will do.

3 The size of rope determines the *size* of cleat. Obviously you want to use the smallest cleat that will hold the rope adequately, so take the rope to the shop and experiment.

4 Some cleats need a *lead*. Work out what your natural sailing position will be when the cleat is used, then mount it at the best angle for jamming. (Most cleats come with plastic wedges, and you can pile them on top of each other to give a variety of 'rakes'.)

With the cleat in the right position for jamming, look where the rope is coming from and decide if you need a lead to guide it in. Remember: if you have to move the tail around when unjammed, as with the mainsheet, then a lead is unwise.

Blocks

A good block changes the lead of a rope with the minimum of friction. In the bad old days large blocks were needed because the size of the bearings determined their efficiency. Now, with ball-bearing blocks, the size can be reduced dramatically. If you can afford it, use ball-bearing blocks wherever there is a load and where the system needs to work well. As with cleats, correct positioning of blocks is vital.

1 Tape the block in position.

2 Put the line in and see if the lead is OK.

3 Only bolt on the block when it works properly. If you can't get it to work, consider mounting the block on an eye so it can float, then use tape or a spring to support it in a central position.

4 Only use a swivel when it is really necessary, because it can twist and cause the rope to rub on itself.

Ratchet blocks act both as a brake and as a cleat. They are only needed on main and genoa sheets, or possibly the sheets of a large spinnaker.

Screws and bolts

Always use stainless screws and bolts – the aluminium variety are not strong enough. Stainless will not cause excessive electrolysis with anodised aluminium fittings.

If there is a substantial load on a fitting, use a bolt rather than a screw. If you can't get behind

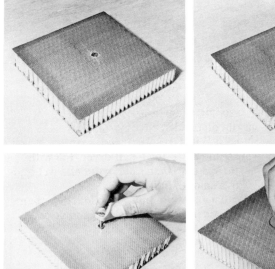
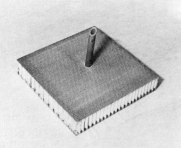
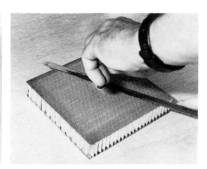
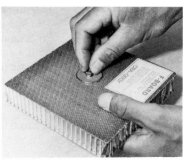

To bolt through honeycomb, first insert a metal spacer tube (to prevent the sides being pulled together).

to fit the nut, consider fitting a hatch, or beefing up the area so you can at least use a hefty screw.

Always use a spring washer under each nut, and do use the right length bolt (or hacksaw off the unwanted end).

Attaching fittings to wood. My preference is for a stainless self-tapper (giving maximum length of thread) with a nylon wing nut on the end. The size of the screw will be determined by the hole in the fitting. (Don't drill out the fitting because it weakens it.)
1 Drill an undersize hole in the wood.
2 Put silicone in the hole, on the screw and on the underside of the fitting.
3 Screw in.

Attaching fittings to glassfibre. Glass is not strong enough to hold fittings on its own: it needs a backing plate of ply.
1 Tape the fitting in place.
2 Drill through, using a slightly undersize drill.
3 Position a varnished ply plate behind the glassfibre.
4 Drill through the ply, too.
5 Put wet varnish on the nut (or on the wing nut if using a self-tapper). This will glue it to the ply when dry, so if you take the fitting off the nut will stay put.
6 Attach the fitting.

If you can't get behind the glassfibre, build up the thickness on top:
1 Make a wooden pad, roughen the bottom and epoxy it to the glass.
2 Drill undersize holes through the fitting, pad and glass.
3 While the epoxy is still wet, screw in self-tappers to pull the pad onto the glass.
4 When the glue sets unscrew and remove the fitting, put silicone on everything and re-attach.

If a pad won't do, consider a hatch.

Attaching fittings to foam sandwich. If you can get behind, fit a backing plate as above. You will also need a stainless tube to act as a spacer for each bolt through the foam sandwich, otherwise the foam will be compressed when you tighten the nut.

If you can't get behind, a plastic Rawlplug hammered into a hole drilled in the foam sandwich may do – provided there is little load on the fitting. Alternatively, try the Allen key trick mentioned on page 11.

4 Care and maintenance

Having gone to so much trouble to work up your boat, you will want to maintain it in tip-top shape.

Hull

The hull can deteriorate from:
- Rig tension. Only use it when you need to.
- Wave action (i.e. pounding). Not much you can do about this!
- Absorbing water. Wash out the boat with fresh water after every outing. Don't forget to hose inside the tanks if they feel damp, wash the mast and boom and deluge all metal fittings to cut electrolysis. If possible, store the boat under cover.
- A poorly shaped trolley. Adapt the chocks to suit the boat.
- Trailing. Avoid wherever possible. If you must tow the boat, tie it down loosely to a wooden box so that if the trailer bends the boat is not distorted. A better method is to put it on the roof, resting either on the deck (not so important as the bottom), or right way up on padded chocks.
- Knocks. With a wooden hull, wash with fresh water, and dry using a hair dryer. Fill with plastic padding; then sand, paint and wet-and-dry to a smooth finish.
  With a glassfibre hull, wash and dry, then use plastic padding (if needed) and gelcoat. Finally, sand off.

Sails

The sails can deteriorate from:
- Ultraviolet light. Put them away when not in use.
- Flogging. Lower all sails as soon as possible; don't sit with them flapping, or hoist them to dry.
- Salt water. Wash each sail with fresh water to prevent the cloth getting hard due to salt penetrating the fibres. (Washing also prevents mildew because a salty sail never really dries.) Hang up by the luff to dry.

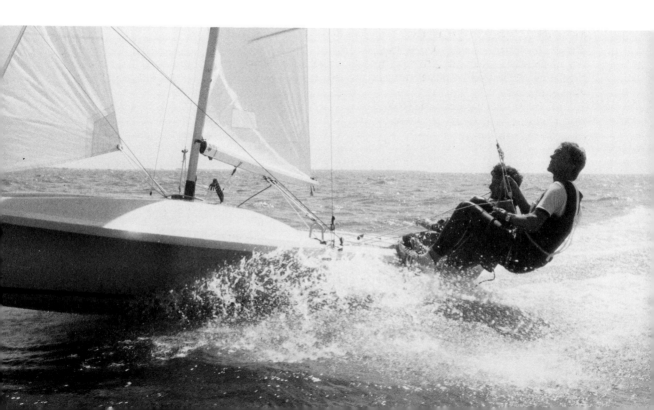

- Creasing. Roll sails rather than fold them.

Foils
The foils can deteriorate from:
- Running aground. A good racing crew is super-careful when landing. Drift ashore as gently as you can, and get the crew over the side early.
- Chipping. When the rudder is not in use, protect it with a padded cover, and make a guard for the trailing edge of the centreboard if it is exposed above the case.

Fittings
Shackles and sheaves may need a squirt of WD40 now and again. But ball-bearing blocks should only be washed with fresh water (no oil or WD40).

Other books in the Sail to Win series

Tactics   *Rodney Pattisson*
A guide to boat-to-boat tactics and strategy around an Olympic course, by gold medallist Rodney Pattisson.

Dinghy Helming   *Lawrie Smith*
One of Britain's top helmsmen gives specific advice on maximising boatspeed in all conditions, plus helming skills required during the race itself.

Dinghy Crewing   *Julian Brooke-Houghton*
Crewing a modern racing dinghy is a complex and demanding task. Olympic medallist Julian Brooke-Houghton explains the skills required and shows how helmsman and crew work together as a race-winning team.

Wind Strategy   *David Houghton*
Most 'sailing weather' books are too large-scale to be relevant to racing on inland or coastal waters. This book shows how to predict the wind over the racecourse area, during the time-span of the race, using simple 'rules of thumb'.

Tuning Your Dinghy   *Lawrie Smith*
A logical, systematic approach to setting up a racing dinghy and fine-tuning it on all points of sailing. Plus a 'trouble shooting' section to pinpoint and cure specific weaknesses in the boat's performance.

The Rules in Practice   *Bryan Willis*
It is a popular fallacy among racing sailors that you need to know the rules. You *do* need to know your rights and obligations on the water – the rules can always be looked up afterwards. International rules experts Bryan Willis looks at the key situations that repeatedly occur on championship courses, from the viewpoint of each helmsman in turn, and summarises what you may, must or cannot do.

Tides and Currents   *David Arnold*
How tides can help you win races – whether inshore, offshore or on an Olympic triangle.